# Air Leak After Pulmonary Resection

*Guest Editor*

ALESSANDRO BRUNELLI, MD

# THORACIC SURGERY CLINICS

www.thoracic.theclinics.com

*Consulting Editor*

MARK K. FERGUSON, MD

August 2010 • Volume 20 • Number 3

SAUNDERS an imprint of ELSEVIER, Inc.

**W.B. SAUNDERS COMPANY**
*A Division of Elsevier Inc.*

1600 John F. Kennedy Boulevard • Suite 1800 • Philadelphia, Pennsylvania 19103-2899

http://www.theclinics.com

**THORACIC SURGERY CLINICS Volume 20, Number 3**
**August 2010 ISSN 1547-4127, ISBN-13: 978-1-4377-1881-2**

Editor: Catherine Bewick

*Thoracic Surgery Clinics* (ISSN 1547-4127) is published quarterly by Elsevier Inc., 360 Park Avenue South, New York, NY 10010-1710. Months of publication are February, May, August, and November. Business and editorial offices: 1600 John F. Kennedy Boulevard, Suite 1800, Philadelphia, PA 19103-2899. Periodicals postage paid at New York, NY, and additional mailing offices. Subscription prices are $269.00 per year (US individuals), $367.00 per year (US institutions), $134.00 per year (US Residents/Students), $343.00 per year (Canadian individuals), $464.00 per year (Canadian institutions), $183.00 per year (Canadian and foreign students), $365.00 per year (foreign individuals), and $464.00 per year (foreign institutions). Foreign air speed delivery is included in all Clinics' subscription prices. All prices are subject to change without notice. **POSTMASTER:** Send address changes to Thoracic Surgery Clinics, Elsevier Health Sciences Division, Subscription Customer Service, 3251 Riverport Lane, Maryland Heights, MO 63043. **Customer Service (orders, claims, online, change of address): Telephone: 1-800-654-2452 (U.S. and Canada); 314-447-8871 (outside U.S. and Canada). Fax: 314-447-8029. Email: journalscustomerservice-usa@elsevier.com (for print support); journalsonlinesupport-usa@elsevier.com (for online support).**

*Reprints.* For copies of 100 or more, of articles in this publication, please contact Commercial Rights Department, Elsevier Inc., 360 Park Avenue South, New York, NY 10010-1710. Tel: (212) 633-3812; Fax: (212) 462-1935; E-mail: reprints@elsevier.com.

*Thoracic Surgery Clinics* is covered in *MEDLINE/PubMed (Index Medicus)* and *EMBASE/Excerpta Medica*.

Printed and bound by CPI Group (UK) Ltd, Croydon, CR0 4YY

Transferred to Digital Print 2012

# Contributors

## CONSULTING EDITOR

**MARK K. FERGUSON, MD**
Professor of Surgery, Section of Cardiac and
Thoracic Surgery, The University of Chicago
Medical Center, Chicago, Illinois

## GUEST EDITOR

**ALESSANDRO BRUNELLI, MD**
Division of Thoracic Surgery, Umberto
I Regional Hospital, Ospedali Riuniti, Ancona,
Italy

## AUTHORS

**S. SCOTT BALDERSON, PA-C**
Department of Surgery, Duke University
Medical Center, Durham, North Carolina

**KEKI R. BALSARA, MD**
Department of Surgery, Duke University
Medical Center, Durham, North Carolina

**EGIDIO BERETTA, MD, PhD**
Department of Experimental Medicine,
Università di Milano-Bicocca, Monza, Italy

**EUGENE H. BLACKSTONE, MD**
Head, Clinical Research, Department
of Thoracic and Cardiovascular Surgery,
Heart and Vascular Institute; Department
of Quantitative Health Sciences, Research
Institute, Cleveland Clinic, Cleveland, Ohio

**ALESSANDRO BRUNELLI, MD**
Division of Thoracic Surgery, Umberto I Regional
Hospital, Ospedali Riuniti, Ancona, Italy

**AYESHA S. BRYANT, MSPH, MD**
Assistant Professor, Division of Cardiothoracic
Surgery, University of Alabama at Birmingham,
Birmingham, Alabama

**STEPHEN D. CASSIVI, MD**
Division of General Thoracic Surgery, Mayo
Clinic, Rochester, Minnesota

**ROBERT J. CERFOLIO, MD, FACS, FCCP**
Professor and Chief of Section of Thoracic
Surgery, Division of Cardiothoracic Surgery;
James H Estes Family Endowed Chair on Lung
Cancer Research, University of Alabama at
Birmingham, Birmingham, Alabama

**GIORGIO F. COLONI, MD**
Department of Thoracic Surgery, University
of Rome SAPIENZA, Rome, Italy

**THOMAS A. D'AMICO, MD**
Professor of Surgery, Department of Surgery,
Duke University Medical Center, Durham,
North Carolina

**MALCOLM M. DECAMP, MD**
Chief, Division of Thoracic Surgery,
Northwestern Memorial Hospital; Professor,
Northwestern University Feinberg School
of Medicine, Chicago, Illinois

**TIZIANO DE GIACOMO, MD**
Department of Thoracic Surgery, University
of Rome SAPIENZA, Rome, Italy

**LISA HALGREN, RN**
Division of General Thoracic Surgery, Mayo
Clinic, Rochester, Minnesota

**MARCELO F. JIMÉNEZ, MD, PhD, FETCS**
Head of Section, Service of Thoracic Surgery, Salamanca University Hospital, Salamanca, Spain

**ADAM LACKEY, MD**
Surgical Resident, Department of Surgery, University of Colorado Denver School of Medicine, Aurora, Colorado

**ROBERT E. MERRITT, MD**
Division of Thoracic Surgery, Department of Cardiothoracic Surgery, Stanford University School of Medicine, Stanford Medical Center, Stanford, California

**GIUSEPPE MISEROCCHI, MD**
Professor of Physiology, Department of Experimental Medicine, Università di Milano-Bicocca, Monza, Italy

**JOHN D. MITCHELL, MD**
Associate Professor of Surgery, Chief, General Thoracic Surgery, Division of Cardiothoracic Surgery, University of Colorado Denver School of Medicine, Aurora, Colorado

**SAILA P. NICOTERA, MD, MPH**
Chief Resident in General Surgery, Department of Surgery, Beth Israel Deaconess Medical Center, Boston, Massachusetts

**NURIA NOVOA, MD, PhD**
Service of Thoracic Surgery, Salamanca University Hospital, Salamanca, Spain

**ERINO A. RENDINA, MD**
Department of Thoracic Surgery, University of Rome SAPIENZA, Rome, Italy

**THOMAS W. RICE, MD**
Head, Thoracic Surgery, Department of Thoracic and Cardiovascular Surgery, Heart and Vascular Institute, Cleveland Clinic, Cleveland, Ohio

**ILARIA RIVOLTA, BD, PhD**
Research Assistant, Department of Experimental Medicine, Università di Milano-Bicocca, Monza, Italy

**GAETANO ROCCO, MD, FRCS (Ed)**
Division of Thoracic Surgery, Department of Thoracic Surgery and Oncology, National Cancer Institute, Pascale Foundation, Naples, Italy

**JOSEPH B. SHRAGER, MD**
Division of Thoracic Surgery, Department of Cardiothoracic Surgery, Stanford University School of Medicine, Stanford Medical Center, Stanford, California; Veterans Affairs Palo Alto Health Care System, Palo Alto, California

**SUNIL SINGHAL, MD**
Division of Thoracic Surgery, Hospital of the University of Pennsylvania, University of Pennsylvania School of Medicine, Philadelphia, Pennsylvania

**GONZALO VARELA, MD, PhD, FETCS**
Head of Service and Professor of Thoracic Surgery, Salamanca University Hospital, Salamanca, Spain

**FEDERICO VENUTA, MD**
Department of Thoracic Surgery, University of Rome SAPIENZA, Rome, Italy

# Contents

Thoracic surgery that requires resection of a portion of lung or of a whole lung profoundly alters the mechanical and fluid dynamic setting of the lung-chest wall coupling, as well as the water balance in the pleural space and in the remaining lung. The most frequent postoperative complications are of a respiratory nature, and their incidence increases the more the preoperative respiratory condition seems compromised. There is an obvious need to identify risk factors concerning mainly the respiratory function, without neglecting the importance of other comorbidities, such as coronary disease. At present, however, a satisfactory predictor of postoperative cardiopulmonary complications is lacking; postoperative morbidity and mortality have remained unchanged in the last 10 years. The aim of this review is to provide a pathophysiologic interpretation of the main respiratory complications of a respiratory nature by relying on new concepts relating to lung fluid dynamics and mechanics. New parameters are proposed to improve evaluation of respiratory function from pre- to the early postoperative period when most of the complications occur.

Practical risk models stratifying the risk of prolonged air leak after pulmonary lobectomy have been developed and discussed. These scores may assist during preoperative patients' counseling, to identify patients at higher risk for prolonged air leak, who may benefit from the use of prophylactic measures such as the use of sealants, buttressed staple lines, or pleural tents. Furthermore, they may be used as standardized inclusion criteria for future randomized clinical trials testing the efficacy of these new technologies, and in doing so make the interpretation of results across different centers and studies more comparable. The clinical use of digital chest drainage units that permit quantitative measurement and recording of air leak flow and intrapleural pressure appears to add to the prediction and management of air leak after pulmonary resection. The use of risk scores based on these digital measures may set the stage for future investigations of active pleural management aimed at treating air leak by tailoring the level of intrapleural pressure to the needs of individual patients.

Thoracoscopic lobectomy has become an accepted, safe, and oncologically sound procedure compared with open lobectomy. Several studies have reported that it reduces the length of stay, postoperative pain, and postoperative complications, including air leaks. Although there are specific technical considerations that must be taken into account, it is increasingly becoming the preferred method of anatomic lobectomy. Surgeons should be encouraged to embrace the minimally invasive strategy, which may be learned in courses using novel simulation techniques. Future directions suggest that this technique will be expanded to address even the most challenging thoracic procedures.

Gaetano Rocco

In thoracic surgery, the intraoperative solution of difficult air space problems relies heavily on the operating surgeon's creativity, versatility, and meticulous surgical technique, as well us profound knowledge of the anatomy and past surgical heritage. The same degree of expertise and experience is needed to simply observe innocent residual spaces without resorting to unnecessary aggressiveness. Management of residual air spaces is an art that conclusively defines the maturity of a thoracic surgeon.

Thomas W. Rice and Eugene H. Blackstone

It is imperative to minimize the occurrence and adverse consequences of air leak complicating pulmonary surgery. This article reviews the contemporary literature and provides recommendations for intraoperative use of agents to control air leak. An evidence-based analysis of the current literature does not support routine use, prophylactically or for air leaks present at operation, of sealants or buttressing material in pulmonary surgery.

Federico Venuta, Erino A. Rendina, Tiziano De Giacomo, and Giorgio F. Coloni

Air leakage after pulmonary resections is considered the most prevalent postoperative problem, and it is often the only morbidity identified. Ideally, treatment begins with prevention; the onset of this complication should be anticipated and recognized during surgery, and intraoperative strategies should be attempted to avoid it and reduce the impact on the clinical course. Once an air leak develops, in most of the cases it seals spontaneously within 2 or 3 days of operation. When it persists, it might elicit the onset of other complications and increase costs and length of hospitalization. The postoperative approaches to a prolonged air leak include management of the pleural drainage and residual space, pleurodesis, pneumoperitoneum, endobronchial one-way valve placement, and potential reoperation.

Robert J. Cerfolio and Ayesha S. Bryant

Most patients who undergo pulmonary resection can have one chest tube and have it removed by postoperative day 3. Air leaks are probably best treated with water seal (passive suction) for most patients with small leaks. If they develop a new or enlarging pneumothorax or subcutaneous emphysema, some suction (active suction) is needed and alternating suction at night with waters seal during the day may be best. Most patients with persistent air leaks can be discharged home safely on an outpatient device and have their tubes removed in 2 to 3 weeks even if they still have an air leak.

> Air leaks after pulmonary resection remain a common occurrence. The impact, or cost, of a complication such as prolonged air leak differs for patients and the involved health care providers. In both cases, the cost is in part determined by the treatment strategy chosen to deal with the complication. Complication costs extend beyond financial aspects and involve quality and delivery of care, postoperative quality of life, and patient satisfaction.

> Recently, several companies have manufactured and commercialized new pleural drainage units that incorporate electronic components for the digital quantification of air through chest tubes and, in some instances, pleural pressure assessment. The goal of these systems is to objectify this previously subjective bedside clinical parameter and allow for more objective, consistent measurement of air leaks. The belief is this will lead to quicker and more accurate chest tube management. In addition, some systems feature portable suction devices. These may afford earlier mobilization of patients because the pleural drainage chamber is attached to a battery-powered smart suction device. In this article we review the clinical experiences using these new devices.

> Ambulatory treatment of pleural problems such as pneumothorax and malignant pleural effusions has been extensively described and is commonly used. On the contrary, outpatient management of chest tubes after lung resection is less frequently performed. Because prolonged air leak after lobectomy is a common problem, early discharge of these patients under pleural drainage can avoid many hospital days without compromising the quality of care. In this article, general rules for outpatient chest tube management are described and available portable devices are reviewed.

> Patients undergoing lung volume reduction surgery and those supported by mechanical ventilation are among our most vulnerable patients. Prolonged air leak in these fragile patients can have dire, even fatal, consequences. This article describes the incidence of prolonged air leak in these populations, the causes ascribed to their development, and strategies that may be applied to their prevention and treatment.

> The management of postoperative alveolar air leaks (AALs) continues to challenge thoracic surgeons. AALs increase length of stay and health care costs, and likely lead to other postoperative complications. Staple line buttresses, topical sealants, pleural tents, pneumoperitoneum, and modifications of traditional chest tube

management (ie, reduced suction) have all been proposed to help reduce AAL. However, the cost of some of the commercial products being marketed may outweigh their relative effectiveness, and some of these techniques and products have not been adequately studied to date. This article provides a review of the available evidence-based literature that addresses the efficacy of the options currently available to prevent and manage AALs. Management suggestions based on this literature are presented.

# Thoracic Surgery Clinics

**THE CLINICS ARE NOW AVAILABLE ONLINE!**

Access your subscription at:
**www.theclinics.com**

# Preface
# Air Leak After Pulmonary Resection

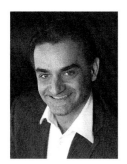

Alessandro Brunelli, MD
*Guest Editor*

Despite recent progress in surgical technique and improved perioperative care, prolonged air leak remains a frequent complication after pulmonary resection. Several studies have shown that air leak and in general chest tube management are the major factors influencing duration of hospital stay and postoperative costs.

This issue of *Thoracic Surgery Clinics* is devoted to the prevention and management of air leak after pulmonary surgery. A preliminary overview of the physics and dynamics of the pleural space is provided in the first article to put in context all the preventative measures or treatments discussed in the following articles. In particular, the relationships between intrapleural pressure, intrapulmonary and pleural fluid filtration, and lung reexpansion are discussed in detail. The concept of passive suction versus active suction applied to chest tubes is also introduced to explain the negative pressure exerted by gravity in contrast to the one applied by external pumps.

The next article focuses on risk factors of prolonged air leak. Different risk scores are provided that can assist clinicians and researchers to stratify the risk of prolonged air leak in lung resection candidates. The subsequent articles discuss different measures that can be used to prevent or treat this complication: surgical techniques, such as the fissureless lobectomy; intraoperative measures, such as pleural tent or pneumoperitoneum; use of sealants or buttressing material; and postoperative rescue strategies, such as blood patching, chemical pleurodesis, or use of endobronchial valves.

The second part of the volume is dedicated to the postoperative management of chest tube, with a particular emphasis on the use of new digitalized systems and portable devices that have the potential to streamline and standardize postoperative practice and facilitate fast-track policies. One article is dedicated to the occurrence and management of air leak in special situations, such as patients with end-stage emphysema submitted to lung volume reduction surgery or those mechanically ventilated. The final article appropriately wraps up this issue of *Thoracic Surgery Clinics* summarizing in an evidence-based format the different treatment options in the management of air leak.

I hope the outstanding contributions collected in this issue will be valuable information that can be used in daily clinical practice and form the basis of future investigations.

Alessandro Brunelli, MD
Division of Thoracic Surgery
Umberto I Regional Hospital, Ospedali Riuniti
Ancona 60020, Italy

E-mail address:
brunellialex@gmail.com

Thorac Surg Clin 20 (2010) xi
doi:10.1016/j.thorsurg.2010.04.005
1547-4127/10/$ – see front matter © 2010 Elsevier Inc. All rights reserved.

# Respiratory Mechanics and Fluid Dynamics After Lung Resection Surgery

Giuseppe Miserocchi, MD*, Egidio Beretta, MD, PhD,
Ilaria Rivolta, BD, PhD

**KEYWORDS**

- Lung edema • Hydrothorax • Air leak
- Lung interstitial pressure • Overdistension

## PROLOGUE: ACTIVE AND PASSIVE DRAINAGE OF THE PLEURAL CAVITY

Postoperative thoracic surgery poses the problem of draining the pleural cavity after closure of the thorax. Two phases in the draining process can be identified. Immediately after closure of the chest, there is a need to drain air to allow lung expansion and volume oscillation during the breathing cycle. Gas drainage ought to be performed by having the tip of the chest tube where the gas bubble is going to collect during the suction process, namely in the less dependent portion of the chest (the retrosternal region in supine posture). As discussed further in the text, complete gas removal is a major cause of over distension for the remaining lung and, in turn, this may represent the pathophysiologic basis common to the 3 main postoperative respiratory complications: air leak, hydrothorax and lung edema. The risk of over distension increases, of course, with increasing the amount of resected lung volume. To prevent the risk of over distension an analysis is presented to provide indications on which suction pressure can be recommended to set a transpulmonary pressure comparable with the preoperative one. This analysis is strongly based on the knowledge of the preoperative elastic characteristics of the patient's lung.

Another indication is that, to avoid over distension, a gas bubble has to remain in the chest in the immediate postoperative period.

After the initial gas drainage, the pressure in the bubble tends to decrease and gas will be progressively replaced by pleural fluid. The amount of pleural fluid being produced reflects the surgical insult and/or an increase in permeability of the mesothelial membranes. Therefore, in this second phase, hydrothorax can develop, which again poses the question of an adequate draining strategy. Because hydrothorax collects in the lowermost part of the pleural space, namely the costodiaphragmatic sinus,[1,2] now the chest tube should drain from the lowermost site of the pleural space. The pressure of the pleural fluid in the costodiaphragmatic sinus is around zero in physiologic conditions, and may become positive with increasing liquid pooling.

**Fig. 1** schematically depicts passive methods to drain the hydrothorax through a chest tube simply sealed under water. By aid of the syringe and a 3-way stopcock, the tube can be filled with fluid (saline solution) to siphon fluid from the chest to the reservoir. Note that the tip of the tube within the chest and the level of the water in the flask are at exactly the same height. Because the pressure acting on the water in the flask is atmospheric, fluid automatically drains into the

Studies reported in this review have been sponsored by funding from Italian Ministry of University, University Milano-Bicocca, ASI (Agenzia Spaziale Italiana).

Department of Experimental Medicine, Università di Milano-Bicocca, Via Cadore 48, Monza 20052, Italy
* Corresponding author.
*E-mail address:* giuseppe.miserocchi@unimib.it

Thorac Surg Clin 20 (2010) 345–357
doi:10.1016/j.thorsurg.2010.03.001
1547-4127/10/$ – see front matter. Published by Elsevier Inc.

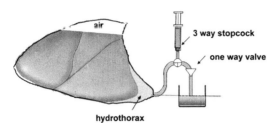

**"PASSIVE DRAINAGE"**
fluid collecting in the lowermost site of cavity will drain
when its pressure exceeds atmospheric pressure

**Fig. 1.** Model of passive pleural fluid drainage from the chest tube placed in the lowermost site of the costodiaphragmatic sinus. By aid of the syringe and a three-way stopcock, the tubing is filled with saline solution to siphon fluid from the chest to the reservoir. The tip of the tube within the chest and the level of the water in the flask are at exactly the same height. Because the pressure acting on the water in the flask is atmospheric, fluid automatically drains into the reservoir whenever the pressure in the hydrothorax exceeds atmospheric pressure. A one-way valve on the tube avoids suction of liquid/air back into the pleural cavity when a subatmospheric pressure is developed on inspiration.

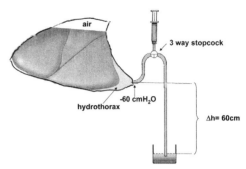

**"ACTIVE DRAINAGE"**
Lowering the bottle with a liquid filled column applies a negative pressure
to the pleural fluid: in this case -60 cmH$_2$O (no one-way valve is needed)

**Fig. 2.** Model of active pleural fluid drainage. Lowering the collecting flask below the tip of the tube (in this case 60 cm), generates a subatmospheric pressure in the chest equal to −60 cm H$_2$O. In this case, pleural fluid is being drained out actively through an increased pressure gradient. No one-way valve is needed for such a negative pressure. Any suction pressure can be generated by adjusting the height of the flask relative to the tip of the chest tube.

reservoir whenever the pressure in the hydrothorax exceeds atmospheric pressure. A one-way valve on the tube avoids suction of liquid/air back into the pleural cavity when a subatmospheric pressure is developed on inspiration.

**Fig. 2** depicts the concept of active drainage. In a fluid-filled system, lowering the collecting flask below the tip of the tube, in this case 60 cm, by putting the flask on the floor with the patient lying in bed, will generate a subatmospheric pressure in the chest of −60 cm H$_2$O. In this case, pleural fluid is being actively drained out down an increased pressure gradient. No one-way valve is needed for such a negative pressure. Any suction pressure can therefore be generated by adjusting the height of the flask relative to the tip of the chest tube. A similar fluid dynamic condition can be maintained by a suitable suction device where setting of the suction pressure is possible.

An active drainage setting of a subatmospheric pressure in the lowermost site of the chest (where the physiologic liquid pressure is basically zero) definitely results in an increase in pleural liquid filtration rate. In this respect, a suction pressure of −60 cm H$_2$O seems incredibly high. Note that the volume of the hydrothorax reflects, over time, the balance between chest drainage and increased pleural filtration rate; shortly after applying the suction pressure, the volume of the hydrothorax might decrease although it keeps increasing again at a later time because of

increased fluid filtration into the pleural cavity. The final volume of the postoperative residual pleural space is determined by the absorption pressure of the pleural lymphatics; this stresses the importance of applying an adequate draining strategy.

## MECHANICS

Thoracic surgery that requires resection of a portion of lung or of a whole lung profoundly alters the mechanical and fluid dynamic setting of the lung-chest wall coupling, as well as the water balance in the pleural space and in the remaining lung. The most frequent postoperative complications are of a respiratory nature, and their incidence increases the more the preoperative respiratory condition seems compromised.[3] There is an obvious need to identify risk factors concerning mainly the respiratory function, without neglecting the importance of other comorbidities, such as coronary disease. At present, however, a satisfactory predictor of postoperative cardiopulmonary complications is still lacking, considering that postoperative morbidity and mortality have remained unchanged in the last 10 years.

The aim of this review is to provide a pathophysiologic interpretation of the main respiratory complications by relying on new concepts relating to lung fluid dynamics and mechanics. New parameters are proposed to improve the evaluation of the respiratory function from pre- to the early postoperative period when most of the complications occur.

### How Lung Expansion is Maintained in the Chest in Physiologic Conditions

It is a common sense to say that a subatmospheric pleural pressure (Ppl) at functional residual capacity results from lung and chest wall exerting a recoil pressure in the opposite direction. Although this statement is correct, it does not say anything about the mechanism responsible for keeping the pleural space free of fluid and gas. Knowledge of this mechanism and its operational features is important to understand how a new equilibrium in the lung-chest wall coupling is being reached after lung resection. The subatmospheric pressure of the pleural fluid reflects the dynamic equilibrium established between the powerful draining action of lymphatics in the face of a low permeability of the filtering mesothelium.[4] This pressure is actually more subatmospheric than the opposite recoil pressure exerted by the lung and chest wall and therefore keeps the visceral and the parietal pleura in close apposition with virtually negligible volume of pleural fluid (0.2 mL/kg).[5,6] Yet, the parietal and visceral pleura do not reciprocally touch (**Fig. 3**) because of repulsive forces acting between polar phospholipids adsorbed on the opposing visceral and parietal membranes.[7] This biochemical setting also guarantees an efficient lubrication system[7] for the reciprocal movement of the pleurae, estimated at about 25,000 km in a life time.

The lymphatic draining system originates at the level of the stomata of the parietal pleura; these are openings 0.3 to 40 μm in diameter, either single or in clusters, directly connecting the pleural space with the submesothelial lymphatic network,[8] they are particularly developed on the diaphragmatic and mediastinal surface. The whole turnover of pleural fluid, ~0.2 mL/(kg × h),[9] is fully regulated at the parietal level as lymphatic absorption sets a liquid pressure causing fluid filtration across the parietal pleura. The visceral pleura is essentially excluded from pleural fluid turnover in physiologic conditions because its permeability is at least 10-fold lower compared with that of the parietal pleura.[10,11] Complete renewal of pleural fluid occurs in about 1 h.

There is an intrapleural liquid circulation (**Fig. 4**) from filtration sites, mostly located in the less dependent portions of the cavity, to the draining regions, mostly located on the diaphragmatic and on the mediastinal surfaces.[4] Pleural fluid protein concentration averages ~1.5 g/dL, indicating a low permeability of the mesothelium for plasma proteins.

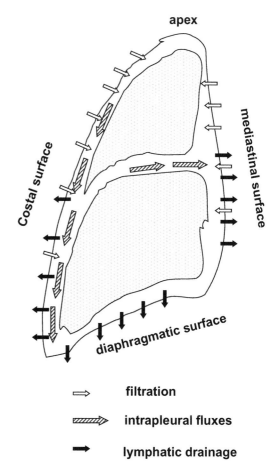

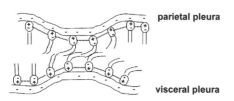

parietal pleura

visceral pleura

⊕ phospholipid molecules adsorbed on mesothelial surface
—— hydrophobic palmitic chains
.......... hydrogen bonds between phospholipid molecules

**Fig. 3.** Model of reciprocal pleural sliding: repulsive forces between several layers of phospholipids adsorbed on mesothelial surfaces carrying charges of the same sign prevent actual touching between opposing pleurae and represent an efficient lubrication system. (*Modified from* Miserocchi G. Mechanisms controlling the volume of pleural fluid and extravascular lung water. Eur Respir Rev 2009;18:244–52; with permission from European Respiratory Society Journals Ltd.)

⇒ **filtration**

⇛ **intrapleural fluxes**

➡ **lymphatic drainage**

**Fig. 4.** Polarization of filtration/drainage processes and of intrapleural fluxes in the pleural cavity. (*Modified from* Miserocchi G. Mechanisms controlling the volume of pleural fluid and extravascular lung water. Eur Respir Rev 2009;18:244–52; with permission from European Respiratory Society Journals Ltd.)

Lymphatics also act as an efficient negative feedback system to regulate pleural fluid dynamics as they can markedly increase draining flow in response to increased filtration.[5]

Pleural liquid pressure varies with height and location within the pleural cavity, as a result of the effect of gravity and intrapleural fluid circulation.[4]

### How Lung Expansion is Altered by Thoracotomy and Lung Resection: the Emphysematous and the Fibrotic Lung

The pleural liquid layer represents a rigid link between chest wall and lung so that changes in chest volume imposed by the action of respiratory muscles are faithfully followed by the lung.

**Fig.** 5A shows the volume-pressure relationships of the lung and chest wall in physiologic conditions and point E, at the crossing between

the 2 curves, corresponds to functional residual capacity (FRC): at this volume, the lung and chest wall exert a recoil pressure equal, but opposite in sign, resulting in a pleural pressure of approximately 6.5 cm $H_2O$. In this plot (Campbell diagram), lung recoil pressure is presented as a negative value, which allows respiratory mechanics to be discussed considering only pleural pressures.

Since the time when Hector was hit in the thorax by Achilles, it is known that, on opening the chest, pneumothorax occurs; as a result, the chest wall expands up to a volume indicated by A (resting point of the chest) and the lung collapses down to minimum volume (resting point of the lung, point B). To save Hector from acute respiratory failure, his chest should have been sutured and a drain placed to clear the pleural cavity from gas; looking at **Fig.** 5A, complete removal of the gas bubble occurs when the distending pressure of the lung

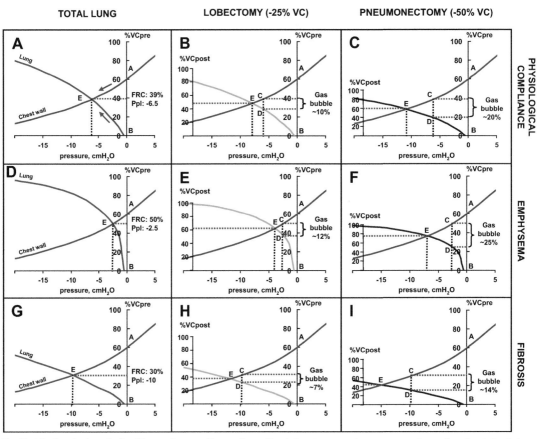

**Fig. 5.** Mechanical analysis of lung-chest wall coupling after lobectomy and pneumonectomy for physiologic lung compliance (A, B, C), increased lung compliance (emphysema, D, E, F) and decreased lung compliance (fibrosis, G, H, I). It is assumed that thoracotomy does not change chest wall compliance and lobectomy and pneumonectomy cause 25% and 50% decrease in lung volume, respectively. The ordinates on the right refer to lung volumes expressed as % of preoperative VC; the ordinates on the left refer to lung volumes expressed as % of postoperative VC.

(Ppl at midheart level) is brought to approximately $-6.5$ cm $H_2O$ (point E). The situation is more complex when lung excision is performed, and the 3 rows in **Fig. 5** show how chest wall-lung mechanical coupling is altered, relative to preoperative conditions, for a lung displaying physiologic compliance (top row), increased lung compliance (emphysema, middle row) and decreased lung compliance (fibrosis, lower row). The cases of lobectomy and pneumonectomy, causing 25% and 50% decrease in vital capacity (VC), respectively, are discussed. Note that the ordinate on the right refers to lung volumes expressed as % of preoperative VC; the ordinate on the left refers to lung volumes expressed as % of postoperative VC. We ignore the elastic properties of the chest wall after thoracotomy, as well as those of a deformed lung, as data are not available in the literature.

**Fig. 5**B refers to lobectomy with physiologic lung compliance; setting drainage to bring Ppl to approximately $-6.5$ cm $H_2O$ clearly implies that the volume of the chest (point C) remains higher than the volume of the lung (point D); the difference C–D represents the volume occupied by gas in the pleural cavity. Decreasing Ppl to about $-7.5$ cm $H_2O$ would allow complete drainage of the gas bubble and close apposition of lung to chest (point E); this implies some over distension of the remaining lung as its FRC would increase to 45% of postoperative VC.

**Fig. 5**C shows the case of pneumonectomy with physiologic lung compliance. Again, points C and D allow estimation of the entity of the gas bubble for a Ppl equal to approximately $-6.5$ cm $H_2O$. Further drainage to reduce the gas bubble to zero (hypothetical point E) to adapt the remaining lung to the whole available volume, would imply major lung deformations, which have never been evaluated. In the hypothetical case of reaching point E, the new FRC would increase to 60% of postoperative VC, a condition clearly representing marked over distension of the remaining lung (Ppl about $-12$ cm $H_2O$).

In **Fig. 5**D presents the case of an emphysematous lung with low recoil pressure (Ppl about $-2.5$ cm $H_2O$); FRC is now increased ($\sim$50% of VC) relative to a lung with normal compliance. After lobectomy (**Fig. 5**E), only a mild suction can bring the remaining lung to the preoperative Ppl (about $-2.5$ cm $H_2O$); furthermore, complete gas drainage (point E) may be obtained by decreasing Ppl to approximately $-3.5$ cm $H_2O$, implying, however, over distension of the remaining lung as postoperative FRC is greater than 60% of postoperative VC. **Fig. 5**F shows that, in case of pneumonectomy, for a Ppl equal to the preoperative

value (about $-2.5$ cm $H_2O$) the volume of the gas bubble would be doubled and its complete removal would cause extreme over distension and deformation of the remaining lung as postoperative FRC would approach $\sim$80% of postoperative VC, with a mild subatmospheric Ppl value.

**Fig. 5**G shows that in a fibrotic lung, FRC is decreased down to 30% of VC, caused by increased lung recoil (about $-10$ cm $H_2O$). Setting this preoperative Ppl after lobectomy and pneumonectomy (see **Fig. 5**H, I, respectively), would imply a smaller gas bubble. In the case of pneumonectomy, the volume of the lung is reduced to become equal to that of the gas bubble. In general, over distension of the remaining lung does not occur in the case of fibrosis.

## How the Work of Breathing is Modified After Lung Resection

Chest wall and lung possess elastic properties, therefore pressure has to be exerted by respiratory muscles on inspiration. The respiratory work may be obtained as:

$$W = \frac{1}{C}V_T^2 \times f$$

where $C$ is lung compliance, $V_T$ is the tidal volume and $f$ is the respiratory frequency. Graphically, respiratory work can be depicted on the volume-pressure curve of the lung by drawing the volume-pressure loops derived from volume-pleural (esophageal) pressure data gathered during the breathing cycle. **Fig. 6**A–C present hypothetical volume-pressure loops. One can appreciate that, for a $V_T$ equal to that in physiologic conditions (20% of preoperative VC), respiratory work increases, as a result of the decrease in lung compliance after lobectomy and pneumonectomy; furthermore, as more subatmospheric Ppl values are generated at end inspiration, this increases the risk of over distension of the remaining lung, the risk being highest after pneumonectomy in emphysematous lung.[12]

The pattern of breathing is actually controlled to minimize its energy cost and this can explain why, particularly after pneumonectomy, the respiratory pattern shows a decrease in tidal volume with a corresponding increase in frequency.[13] Considerations concerning the work of breathing become important when evaluating the postoperative working capacity of the patient. Lobectomy has little effect on maximum workload, whereas pneumonectomy results in a 25% decrease.[14] Respiratory and leg fatigue sensation (estimated with the Borg scale) were found to be greater, for the same workload, after pneumonectomy.[14] There

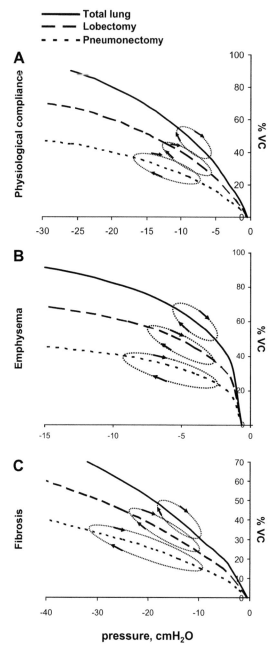

**Fig. 6.** Hypothetical volume-pressure loops to depict respiratory work on the volume-pressure relationships of the preoperative lung, after lobectomy and pneumonectomy for physiologic (*A*), increased (emphysema, *B*) and decreased (fibrosis, *C*) lung compliance. Inspiratory and expiratory pressures are indicated by upward and downward directed arrows, respectively.

are indications that after lobectomy, exercise capacity is, like in healthy people, limited by leg fatigue, whereas after pneumonectomy it is limited by respiratory fatigue and dyspnea.[13]

## LUNG WATER BALANCE
### Lung Fluid Balance and Tissue Mechanics in Physiologic Conditions

The pressure existing in the interstitial space of the lung is subatmospheric,[16] about $-10$ cm $H_2O$, reflecting, as much as for the pleural space, a strong draining lymphatic action, in the face of a low permeability of the capillary endothelium providing fluid filtration (**Fig. 7**). A subatmospheric interstitial pressure keeps the endothelium well glued to the epithelium, and in this way the volume of the extravascular water is kept at a minimum so that the overall thickness of the air-blood barrier is approximately 0.5 µm. The lung strongly resists conditions that cause an increase in microvascular filtration, potentially causing edema,[16] as several mechanisms cooperate to allow minimal variations in the volume of the extravascular water. A key role is played by proteoglycans, a family of compounds that act as link molecules within the extracellular matrix and between the capillary and the alveolar walls. Proteoglycans, through their glycosaminoglycan chains, can bind excess water in the interstitial space to form gel-like structures. Furthermore, through their macromolecular assembly, they confer low compliance to the interstitial compartment; as shown in **Fig. 8**, in response to increased filtration, a minor increase in extravascular water ($\sim 10\%$) causes an increase in interstitial pressure by about 15 cm $H_2O$ (from $-10$ to 5 cm $H_2O$,

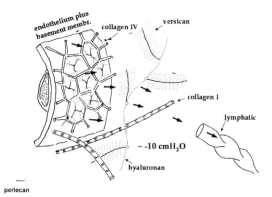

**Fig. 7.** The physiologic fluid turnover in the lung interstitium. A subatmospheric interstitial pressure results from the balance between the absorption pressure of lymphatics and microvascular filtration through a low permeability endothelial barrier. Some important molecules of the extracellular matrix are indicated. (*From* Miserocchi G. Lung interstitial pressure and structure in acute hypoxia. In: Roach R, Wagner PD, Hackett P, editors. Hypoxia and the circulation. Advances in experimental medicine and biology, vol. 618. New York: Springer; 2007. p. 141–57, Fig. 4; with kind permission of Springer Science and Business Media.)

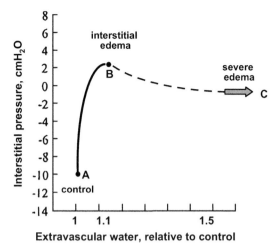

**Fig. 8.** The continuous line shows the time course of lung interstitial pressure when interstitial edema develops (point A to point B); note the marked increase in interstitial pressure for a minor change in extravascular water reflecting the very low compliance of the lung interstitial matrix. The dashed line shows the time course of interstitial pressure when severe edema develops (point B to point C); the decrease in pressure reflects the loss of integrity of the macromolecular structure of the extracellular matrix caused by fragmentation of proteoglycans that results in increase in tissue compliance and in microvascular permeability. Restoring the filtration gradient leads to unopposed filtration and to severe edema (*arrow*). (*Modified from* Miserocchi G. Mechanisms controlling the volume of pleural fluid and extravascular lung water. Eur Respir Rev 2009;18:244–52; with permission from European Respiratory Society Journals Ltd.)

a continuous line from point A to B)[16]: the marked increase in interstitial pressure buffers further filtration (so-called tissue safety factor).

### How Lung Fluid Balance may be Altered by Lung Resection: the Idiopathic Lung Edema

Pulmonary complications represent the most frequent cause of morbidity and mortality in the postoperative period. Despite different clinical manifestation identified as edema, acute lung injury, atelectasis, acute respiratory distress syndrome, the common physiopathologic mechanism underlying these complications is a severe perturbation in lung water balance. In spite of a remarkable resistance of the lung to developing edema, several cofactors may acutely induce an increase in microvascular filtration[16] following lung resection. The sequence of events leading to the increase in extravascular lung water are important.[16] There is experimental proof that severe lung edema develops acutely when the

lung interstitial pressure decreases, as indicated by C in **Fig. 8**; this restores a pressure gradient to cause unopposed fluid filtration from the capillaries toward the interstitial compartment and the alveoli. The reason for the decrease in interstitial pressure is the loss of integrity of the native architecture of the proteoglycans of the interstitial matrix and of the basement membrane[16] leading to an increase in tissue compliance and in microvascular permeability. Beyond a critical threshold in the process of fragmentation, the combination of these 2 effects leads to the accelerated phase of development of severe lung edema.[16] The causes for a loss of integrity of the proteoglycan matrix include weakening of their linking noncovalent chemical bonds caused by hydration, increase in parenchymal stresses, and activation of tissue metalloproteases.[16] These pathophysiologic mechanisms are common to all forms of lung edema, the only difference being the sequence of proteoglycans fragmentation. In the so-called hydraulic edema (as in left heart failure) the fragmentation process initially involves the large matrix proteoglycans of the matrix; in the permeability type of edema (as in acute pancreatitis) there is a major initial degradation of proteoglycans of the basement membrane. Tissue hypoxia is another known cause of lung edema with features that are intermediate between the hydraulic and the permeability type.[17] Thus, there may be a variable contribution to edema formation due either to the loss of tissue safety factor or to an increase in microvascular permeability. In general, interstitial lung edema ought to be considered as a sharp edge between tissue repair and manifestation of a severe disease. Tissue remodeling was triggered in response to increased microvascular filtration by signaling transduction initiated within 3 hours in endothelial and epithelial cells during interstitial lung edema.[18–21] Matrix turnover reflects the critical balance between fragmentation and deposition and it is therefore important to review the conditions favoring edema formation, as they may coexist in the early postoperative period:

- After lung resection the same cardiac output flows through a decreased vascular bed. Because a minor increase in pulmonary artery pressure has been reported, this suggests that pulmonary capillary recruitment has occurred, thus increasing the overall microvascular filtration surface area favoring lung edema.
- An increase in blood volume and flow velocity in the lung microcirculation increases the endothelial shear stress,[22]

an important cofactor leading to increase in microvascular permeability. A pathophysiologic mechanism leading to lung edema based on over perfusion explains the finding that inhaled NO, proposed to prevent postpneumonectomy pulmonary edema, actually worsened the case.[23]

- Local hypoxia[17,24] may occur in a postoperative diseased lung. A $P_{O_2}$ falling below about 40 mm Hg was shown to trigger the activation of tissue metalloproteases that cause fragmentation of proteoglycans.[16,17] Hypoxia is known to cause precapillary vasoconstriction. Although the specific role of this response is not fully understood, it is suggested that this avoids an increase in capillary pressure in a condition of increased microvascular filtration. So, on the one hand, local hypoxia favors edema formation by triggering extravascular matrix degradation; on the other hand it limits microvascular filtration avoiding an increase in capillary perfusion pressure. The balance between these 2 effects is difficult to predict. A fully oxygenated blood (possibly hyperoxic) after lung resection would certainly cause full recruitment of the microvascular bed that, per se, is a cause of increased microvascular filtration. Possibly, this condition might be buffered through a mild degree of blood de-oxygenation sufficient to evoke precapillary vasoconstriction without triggering the action of metalloproteases.
- Fragmentation of the extracellular matrix and lack of clearance of the fragments is involved in neutrophil activation.[25] Neutrophil activation leads to production of reactive oxygen species causing a major increase in microvascular permeability, diffuse alveolar damage, and inhibition of the active alveolar fluid reabsorption.[26] There is evidence that removal of matrix fragments is critical for successful repair[27]; in particular failure to clear hyaluronan fragments leads to unremitting inflammation.[28]

Other important cofactors that favor postpneumonectomy idiopathic lung edema formation are:

- Over inflation caused by aggressive drainage to force the apposition between lung and chest or caused by prolonged mechanical ventilation with excessive tidal volume[29]: retrospective studies have recognized these conditions as cofactors of lung edema.[30–32] The underlying

physiologic mechanism in both cases is exactly the same: stretching of lung parenchyma results in a marked subatmospheric interstitial pressure, that, in turn, favors microvascular filtration,[30] the first step toward the development of edema.

- Large amounts of intraoperative fluid administered as originally reported by Zeldin and colleagues[33] and recently resumed by Slinger[34]: there are considerable interindividual differences in the resistance of the lung to edema formation.

## CLINICAL CONSIDERATIONS
### The Postoperative Residual Pleural Space

As described in the analysis of **Fig. 5**, complete gas removal is a major cause of lung over distension that in turn leads to the 3 main postoperative respiratory complications: air leak, hydrothorax, and lung edema. To avoid over distension, a gas bubble has to remain in the chest in the immediate postoperative period after placing a suction tube. Gas is slowly reabsorbed ($\sim 1\%$/d) from the chest; washing the cavity with oxygen would speed up the reabsorption process. Within the gas bubble, pressure tends to decrease as a result of equilibration of atmospheric oxygen with its partial pressure in the venous blood; this, in turn, causes an increase in pleural fluid filtration so that, with time, liquid will replace gas. The absorption pressure of the pleural lymphatics determines the volume of the postoperative residual pleural space and the transpulmonary pressure of the deformed remaining lung. The volume of the postoperative residual pleural space is occupied in part by pleural fluid, in part by the remaining lung undergoing partial deformation, in part by the displacement of the diaphragm (upward) and of the mediastinum (toward the site of lung resection). A postoperative residual pleural space was diagnosed in more than 90% of the cases of lobectomy[35] and, as detailed in the analysis of **Fig. 5**, the preoperative lung compliance is an important determinant of its final volume. When considering the postoperative residual pleural space:

- in emphysema, lobectomy and pneumonectomy result in over distension of the remaining lung, with low subatmospheric pleural pressures, thus implying a greater risk of air leak.
- in fibrosis, pleural pressures become remarkably subatmospheric exceeding the draining pressure of lymphatics, implying a greater risk for persistency of the gas bubble (potentially misinterpreted as air

leak), and formation of hydrothorax caused by increased fluid filtration.

## The Management of the Chest Tube

An important issue to be considered at this point is that the volume of the postoperative residual pleural space cannot be imposed by the suction pressure, which should actually serve only to help in reaching the new mechanical and fluid dynamic equilibrium at pleural level. The first problem the surgeon faces after closure of the chest is the need to clear gas from the cavity to allow lung expansion and volume oscillation during the breathing cycle. This is probably the most critical part to avoid lung over distension (with the exception of lobectomy in a lung with physiologic compliance). Apparently, no definite protocols are available concerning the initial gas drainage. The analysis of **Fig. 5** might provide useful indications, but implies a more thorough preoperative pneumologic evaluation. A high FRC with a poorly subatmospheric pleural pressure, as measured by an eosphageal balloon (less negative than $-6.5$ cm $H_2O$) indicates emphysema, whereas a decrease in FRC with a subatmospheric pressure substantially more negative than $-6.5$ cm $H_2O$ indicates fibrosis. Setting a suction pressure on the chest tube that restores the preoperative transpulmonary pressure (points C and D in the graphs) certainly avoids over distension; setting a transpulmonary pressure corresponding to point E certainly implies over distension. To monitor transpulmonary pressure after closure of the chest requires the measurement of esophageal pressure (no such data are available in the literature).

An appreciable draining strategy is based on a balanced suction device[36,37] that implies the placement of 2 intrathoracic catheters, one (sealed with water) placed at the base of the lung to drain fluid, the other placed in the apical region to allow air to enter the chest whenever intrapleural pressures generated during inspiration are lower than a preset value (usually $-10$ to $-15$ cm $H_2O$). This strategy assumes that a gas bubble remains in the chest to avoid over distension of the lung. The use of a balanced suction device was reported to reduce the risk of pulmonary edema.[35] To a physiologist, this setting seems fully justified; although, on a clinical level, the use of 2 chest tubes seems more complicated and implies more postoperative pain.[38] Another alternative is to insert in the lower chest only 1 tube with 2 openings, 1 at the tip to reach the gas in the less dependent portion of the cavity, the other at some distance to drain fluid from the bottom of the cavity.[38] This setting allows some recirculation of pleural fluid; whenever the pressure in the gas bubble becomes markedly subatmospheric on inspiration, fluid might be sucked up from the lowermost part of the chest and outflow from the top opening. This method decreases the volume of fluid drained from the cavity and postoperative pain.[38]

### The air leak

A persistent air leak following pulmonary resection may represent a common problem[39] and may arise from a major airway (bronchopleural fistula) or from the most peripheral airways (bronchoalveolar-pleural fistula) because of failure to obtain a perfect intraoperative seal. It has been reported that the surgical approach is not predictive of a persistent air leak. As discussed earlier, the risk of over distension is higher after pneumonecotmy in an emphysematous patient in whom recoil pressure is markedly decreased. It can be hypothesized that the suction pressure of pleural lymphatics may be such as to force the lung against the chest wall, thus considerably reducing the postoperative residual pleural space.

Over distention of the lung is favored at end inspiration; de-stretching of the lung parenchyma during expiration temporarily seals the lung. The risk of air leak on inspiration is greater for the emphysematous lung and, potentially, also for the fibrotic lung as transpulmonary pressures generated are more subatmospheric.

### The hydrothorax

A recent paper[38] proposes the right question concerning the pleural fluid dynamic situation after lung resection: "Is it really necessary to drain all the fluid in pleural space by chest tube or can the pleura absorb this excess fluid physiologically?" On studying experimental hydrothorax[6] the answer is that pleural lymphatics can generate a pressure to bring the lung close to the chest with minimal residual pleural liquid volume. After lung resection this statement still holds true, but the postoperative residual pleural space, as discussed earlier, reflects the complex balance between fluid filtration/lymphatic absorption and chest/lung recoil pressure. Hydrothorax is favored by aggressive management of the chest tube because an excessive subatmospheric pressure may cause an increase in fluid filtration. This condition characteristically occurs if the fluid collecting flask is placed on the floor (see **Fig. 2**). Another cause of hydrothorax is an increase in microvascular permeability of either the parietal or the visceral pleura as a result of postoperative inflammation. Full recovery from pleural effusion caused by increased permeability is a long process even though the lymphatic mechanism is quite adaptive (flow rate can increase by 20/30 times); the time course of this process is critically dependent on restoring a physiologically low mesothelial permeability. Recovery times range from weeks (after myocardial infarction and coronary artery by pass) to months (this is the case for tuberculosis and asbestosis).[40] There is a suggestion that the chest tube should be removed when 450 mL are recovered.[41]

### Preoperative Versus Postoperative Assessment: FEV₁, DLco, Vo₂max

In the presence of some degree of preoperative respiratory deficiency, there is an obvious concern that postoperative impairment of respiratory function might become acutely critical for survival.

The complimentary use of spirometry and lung diffusing capacity have been extensively reviewed in recent articles,[29,42] therefore the authors only refer to specific pathophysiologic issues. In general, these parameters can predict postoperative conditions at 3 to 6 months. However, they do not allow prediction of severe complications that occur in the early postoperative period. Postoperative predicted values largely underestimate the actual decrease observed in this critical period.

Concerning $FEV_1$ measurements, the recognized drawbacks for preoperative risk stratification[42] are:

- preoperative absolute cutoff values, rather than percentage, ignoring differences in gender, age, and body size
- preoperative $FEV_1$ values can lead to inappropriate exclusion of patients[43] and cannot be related to the surgical outcome[44]
- $FEV_1$ is a poor predictor of change in exercise capacity after lung resection.[14]

DLco measurement was highly recommended as an independent strong predictor of postoperative mortality and pulmonary morbidity in patients with or without chronic obstructive pulmonary disease.[45] There is a recommendation to measure DLco routinely as a preoperative evaluation, regardless of the outcome of the spirometric evaluation[29]; a predictive postoperative DLco of less than 40% was proposed as a cutoff for normal and high-risk patients.[29] Poor correlation was found between DLco and $FEV_1$.[46]

Cardiopulmonary exercise testing together with DLco are the best methods to evaluate the efficiency of the whole chain of oxygen delivery. Vo₂max was obviously decreased after lung resection although the reduction was not in proportion to the volume of lung resected.[47] The decrease in Vo₂max was found, on average, to

be much greater than the decrease in DLco,[48] suggesting an additional cardiovascular or metabolic impairment. The use of near-infrared spectroscopy (NIRS)[49] on exercising muscles identifies potential metabolic limitations of the working muscles. NIRS is a noninvasive approach that uses the differential absorption properties of hemoglobin to evaluate skeletal muscle deoxygenated hemoglobin during work, which reflects the metabolic capacity of the muscle.

The decrease in Vo₂max was accompanied by a decrease in cardiac output, an increase in pulmonary artery pressure and in pulmonary vascular resistance.[47]

### The Need for Early Postoperative Assessment

Most of the respiratory complications occur in the early postoperative period.[50] Predicted postoperative values of $FEV_1$ and DLco are not valid predictors of respiratory complications in the immediate postoperative period.[42] Furthermore, available conventional models, based on the number of lung segments removed, underestimate the loss of $FEV_1$ and DLco that occur in the early postoperative period. KCO was found to increase on the first postoperative day, the increase being significantly greater after pneumonectomy compared with lobectomy (15% compared with 2.6%, respectively). This finding requires careful interpretation, particularly because it correlated with a low preoperative DLco. The increase in KCO could be explained by a remarkable increase in pulmonary capillary blood volume (commonly referred to as Vc, a subcomponent of DLco). The increase in Vc is compatible with over perfusion of the remaining lung, which is of greater entity after pneumonectomy. As discussed earlier, pulmonary congestion and over distension are two important comorbidity factors leading to increased microvascular filtration. Under these conditions, adequate clearance of the interstitial fluid is a potent factor preventing lung edema and respiratory movements help the lymphatics in this important draining process.[4] In agreement with this interpretation is the important report[48] that epidural anesthesia, which allows a normal pattern of breathing, reduces postoperative respiratory complications by one-third.

### SUGGESTIONS: HOW TO IMPROVE PRE- TO EARLY POSTOPERATIVE EVALUATION

Because surgeons are attaining considerable technical refinement,[42] there is an obvious need to also refine the identification of risk factors for respiratory distress to reduce morbidity and mortality. The postoperative period seems to be the most critical period, when cofactors of respiratory morbidity may be present.

To prevent over distension, knowledge of the elastic properties of the lung would be useful. To follow the time evolution of the lung fluid balance, 2 methods can be suggested. The first is to measure lung reactance by forced oscillatory technique (FOT) using a frequency of 4 to 5 Hz. This parameter was shown to decrease progressively and significantly with increasing extravascular water volume not exceeding 10%, representing an early and sensitive marker of development of lung edema, before any change in lung compliance can be detected.[51] The method is simple, noninvasive, and does not require the collaboration of the patient. No reference values are provided for the population, therefore, each patient will be their own control from the pre- to postoperative period.

The other method to reveal early perturbation of lung fluid balance is to detect lung comets by chest sonography ultrasound.[52] A lung comet is defined as an echogenic, coherent, wedge-shaped signal with a narrow origin from the hyperechoic pleural line. The total number of comets yields the comet score, which quantifies the increase in extravascular water. This technique has become increasingly popular and is sensitive for detecting the early phase of developing lung edema.

Surgery, mechanical ventilation, and edema formation might decrease surfactant activity[53] at the alveolar level, as indicated by the occurrence of atelectasis. Intratracheal instillation of surfactant is a further possibility.

## SUMMARY
### Respiratory Mechanics

- In emphysema, lobectomy and pneumonectomy result in over distension of the remaining lung, thus implying a greater risk of air leak.
- In fibrosis, pleural pressures become remarkably subatmospheric implying a greater risk for persistence of the gas bubble (potentially misinterpreted as air leak) and formation of hydrothorax.
- Respiratory work increases after lobectomy and pneumonectomy, because lung compliance decreases in inverse proportion to the volume resected.
- The increase in respiratory work after pneumonectomy elicits dyspnea, which limits exercise capacity.

### Lung Fluid Balance

- The common pathophysiologic mechanism underlying the postoperative respiratory complications is a severe perturbation in lung water balance leading to edema.
- Microvascular filtration is increased in the remaining lung by capillary recruitment and by a marked subatmospheric interstitial pressure resulting from stretching of lung parenchyma caused by over distension (due to aggressive drainage or prolonged mechanical ventilation).

### Clinical Considerations

- Complete postoperative gas removal is a major cause of lung over distension that leads to the 3 main respiratory complications: air leak, hydrothorax, and lung edema.
- The postoperative residual pleural space is set by the absorption pressure of the pleural lymphatics; its volume is occupied by pleural fluid, the remaining lung, the displacement of the diaphragm and of the mediastinum.
- Air leak and hydrothorax are favored by an excessive subatmospheric pressure applied to the chest tube.

### Suggestions

- Knowledge of the elastic properties of the lung would be useful to set a pleural pressure that prevents over distension.
- Sensitive markers of developing lung edema in the immediate postoperative phase are the measurement of lung reactance by FOT and detection of lung comets by chest sonography ultrasound.

## REFERENCES

1. Miserocchi G, Negrini D, Pistolesi M, et al. Intrapleural liquid flow down a gravity dependent hydraulic pressure gradient. J Appl Phys 1988;64:577–84.
2. Haber R, Grotberg JB, Glucksberg MR, et al. Steady-state pleural fluid flow and pressure and the effects of lung buoyancy. J Biomech Eng 2001; 123:485–92.
3. Licker M, de Perrot M, Hohn L, et al. Preoperative mortality and major cardiopulmonary complications after lung surgery for non-small carcinoma. Eur J Cardiothorac Surg 1999;5:314–9.
4. Miserocchi G, Negrini D. Pleural space: pressure and fluid dynamics. In: Crystal RG, West JB, editors. The lung: scientific foundations. New York: Raven Press; 1997. p. 1217–25.
5. Miserocchi G, Venturoli D, Negrini D, et al. Model of pleural fluid turnover. J Appl Phys 1993;75(4):1798–806.

6. Miserocchi G. Mechanisms controlling the volume of pleural liquid and extravascular lung water. Eur Respir Rev 2009;18:244–52.

7. Hills BA. Graphite-like lubrication of mesothelium by oligolamollar pleural surfactant. J Appl Phys 1992; 73:1034–9.

8. Wang NS. Anatomy of the pleura. Clin Chest Med 1998;19:229–40.

9. Miserocchi G. Physiology and pathophysiology of pleural fluid turnover. Eur Respir J 1997;10: 219–25.

10. Negrini D, Reed RK, Miserocchi G. Permeability-surface area product and reflection coefficient of the parietal pleura in dogs. J Appl Phys 1991;71:2543–7.

11. Negrini D, Townseley MI, Taylor AE. Hydraulic conductivity and osmotic reflection coefficient of canine parietal pleura in vivo. J Appl Phys 1994; 76:627–33.

12. McIlroy MB, Bates DV. Respiratory function after pneumonectomy. Thorax 1956;11:303–11.

13. Bolliger CT, Jordan P, Solèr M, et al. Pulmonary function and exercise capacity after lung resection. Eur Respir J 1996;9:415–21.

14. Pelletier C, Lapointe L, LeBlanc P. Effects of lung resection on pulmonary function and exercise capacity. Thorax 1990;45:497–502.

15. Miserocchi G, Negrini D, Gonano C. Direct measurements of interstitial pulmonary pressure in in-situ lung with intact pleural space. J Appl Phys 1990; 69(6):2168–74.

16. Miserocchi G, Negrini D, Passi A, et al. Development of lung edema: interstitial fluid dynamics and molecular structure. News Physiol Sci 2001;16:66–71.

17. Miserocchi G, Passi A, Negrini D, et al. Pulmonary interstitial pressure and tissue matrix structure in acute hypoxia. Am J Physiol Lung Cell Mol Physiol 2001;280:L881–7.

18. Palestini P, Calvi C, Conforti E, et al. Composition, biophysical properties and morphometry of plasma membranes in pulmonary interstitial edema. Am J Physiol Lung Cell Mol Physiol 2002;282:L1382–90.

19. Palestini P, Calvi C, Conforti E, et al. Compositional changes in lipid microdomains of air-blood barrier plasma membranes in pulmonary interstitial edema. J Appl Phys 2003;95:1446–52.

20. Daffara R, Botto L, Beretta E, et al. Endothelial cells as early sensors of pulmonary interstitial edema. J Appl Phys 2004;97(4):1575–83.

21. Botto L, Beretta E, Daffara R, et al. Biochemical and morphological changes in endothelial cells in response to hypoxic interstitial edema. Respir Res 2006;13(7):7.

22. Min-Ho K, Harris NR, Tarbell JM. Regulation of capillary hydraulic conductivity in response to an acute change in shear. Am J Physiol Heart Circ Physiol 2005;289:H2126–35.

23. Filaire M, Fadel E, Decante B, et al. Inhaled nitric oxide does not prevent postpneumonectomy pulmonary edema in pigs. J Thorac Cardiovasc Surg 2007;133:770–4.

24. Hansen J, Olsen N, Feldt-Rasmussen B, et al. Albuminuria and overall capillary permeability of albumin in acute altitude hypoxia. J Appl Phys 1994;76:1922–7.

25. Adair-Kirk TL, Senior RM. Fragments of extracellular matrix as mediators of inflammation. Int J Biochem Cell Biol 2008;40:1101–10.

26. Khimenko PL, Barnard JW, Moore TM, et al. Vascular permeability and epithelial transport effects on lung edema formation in ischemia and reperfusion. J Appl Phys 1994;77(3):1116–21.

27. Teder P, Vandivier RV, Jang D, et al. Resolution of lung inflammation by CD44. Science 2002;296: 155–8. DOI:10.1126/science.1069659.

28. Noble PW, Jiang D. Matrix regulation of lung injury, inflammation, and repair: the role of innate immunity. Proc Am Thorac Soc 2006;3:401–4.

29. Ferguson MK, Lehman AG, Bolliger CT, et al. The role of diffusing capacity and exercise tests. Thorac Surg Clin 2008;18:9–17.

30. Alvarez JM, Tan J, Kejriwal N, et al. Idiopathic postpneumonectomy pulmonary edema: hyperinflation of the remaining lung is a potential etiologic factor, but the condition can be averted by balanced pleural drainage. J Thorac Cardiovasc Surg 2007; 133:1439–47.

31. Fernandez-Pérez ER, Keegan MT, Brown DR, et al. Intraoperative tidal volume as a risk factor for respiratory failure after pneumonectomy. Anesthesiology 2006;105:14–8.

32. Miserocchi G, Negrini D, Gonano C. Parenchymal stress affects interstitial and pleural pressure in in situ lung. J Appl Phys 1991;71:1967–72.

33. Zeldin RA, Normadin D, Landwing BS, et al. Postpenumonectomy pulmonary edema. J Thorac Cardiovasc Surg 1984;87:359–65.

34. Slinger PD. Postpneumonectomy pulmonary edema. Anesthesiology 2006;105:2–5.

35. Misthos P, Kokotsakis J, Konstantinou M, et al. Postoperative residual pleural spaces: characteristics and natural history. Asian Cardiovasc Thorac Ann 2007;15:54–8.

36. Pecora DV, Cooper P. Pleural drainage following pneumonectomy: description of apparatus. Surgery 1955;37:251.

37. Alvarez JM, Panda RK, Newman MA, et al. Postpneumonectomy pulmonary edema. J Cardiothorac Vasc Anesth 2003;17(3):388–95.

38. Okur E, Baysungur V, Tezel C, et al. Comparison of the single or double chest tube applications after pulmonary lobectomies. Eur J Cardiothorac Surg 2009;35:32–6.

39. Rice TW, Okereke IC, Blackstone EH. Persistent airleak following pulmonary resection. Chest Surg Clin N Am 2002;12:529–39.

40. Cohen M, Sahn SA. Resolution of pleural effusions. Chest 2001;119:1547–62.
41. Cerfolio RJ, Bryant AS. Results of a prospective algorithm to remove chest tubes after pulmonary resection with high output. J Thorac Cardiovasc Surg 2008;135:269–73.
42. Brunelli A, Rocco G. Spirometry: predicting risk and outcome. Thorac Surg Clin 2008;18:1–8.
43. Linden PA, Bueno R, Colson YL, et al. Lung resection in patients with preoperative FEV1 <35% predicted. Chest 2005;127:1984–90.
44. Rocco G. Predicting the postoperative outcome after lung surgery. Chest 2001;120:1761.
45. Ferguson MK, Little L, Rizzo L, et al. Diffusing capacity predicts morbidity ad mortality after pulmonary resection. J Thorac Cardiovasc Surg 1988;96:894–900.
46. Brunelli A, Refai M, Salati M, et al. Carbon monoxide lung diffusive capacity improves risk-stratification in patients without flow limitation: evidence for systematic measurement before lung resection. Eur J Cardiothorac Surg 2006;29:567–70.
47. Nezu K, Kushibe K, Takahama M, et al. Recovery and limitation of exercise capacity after lung resection for lung cancer. Chest 1998;113:1511–6.
48. Licker MJ, Widikker I, Robert J, et al. Operative mortality and respiratory complications after lung resection for cancer: impact of chronic obstructive pulmonary disease and time trends. Ann Thorac Surg 2006;81:1830–8.
49. Mancini DM, Bolinger L, Li H, et al. Validation of near-infra-red spectroscopy in humans. J Appl Phys 1994;77(6):2740–7.
50. Varela G, Brunelli A, Rocco G, et al. Evidence of lower alteration of expiratory volume in patients with airflow limitation in the immediate period after lobectomy. Ann Thorac Surg 2007;84(2):417–22.
51. Dellacà RL, Zannin E, Sancini G, et al. Changes in the mechanical properties of the respiratory system during the development of interstitial lung edema. Respir Res 2008;9:51.
52. Picano E, Frassi F, Agricola E, et al. Ultrasound lung comets: a clinically useful sign of extravascular lung water. J Am Soc Echocardiogr 2006;19:356–63.
53. Günther A, Siebert C, Schmidt R, et al. Surfactant alterations in severe pneumonia, acute respiratory distress syndrome, and cardiogenic lung edema. Am J Respir Crit Care Med 1996;153(1):176–84.

# Risk Factors for Prolonged Air Leak After Pulmonary Resection

Alessandro Brunelli, MD[a],*, Stephen D. Cassivi, MD[b], Lisa Halgren, RN[b]

**KEYWORDS**

- Prolonged air leak • Pulmonary lobectomy • Risk models
- Risk factors • Chest drainage • Chest tubes

Air leaks remain a frequent and bothersome complication after pulmonary resection. Their incidence is dependent on many factors, including the physiologic and anatomic characteristics of the patients at the time of surgery and their definition.

Up to 30% to 50% of patients may show evidence of air leak from the chest drain after lobectomy either immediately after the operation or during the first postoperative day.[1–4] This incidence progressively decreases in the subsequent postoperative days. Approximately 8% to 15% of patients ultimately will have what is, by current convention, regarded as a prolonged air leak (PAL).[5,6] It has been shown that PAL may prolong the hospital stay, negatively impacting hospitalization costs,[7–10] increasing the risk of empyema,[10] as well as other possible cardiopulmonary complications.[1,9] Predicting the risk of PAL therefore may assist in adopting prophylactic or therapeutic measures aimed at reducing the occurrence of this complication. During preoperative counseling, patients should be informed about their expected PAL risk and be prepared for the possibility of being discharged from hospital following surgery with a portable chest drainage unit to minimize their length of hospitalization.

Finally, developing reliable risk models that can stratify the risk of PAL may permit selection of patients to be included in prospective randomized trials testing the efficacy of new intraoperative or postoperative devices or technologies aimed at reducing the incidence of PAL.

## DEFINITION OF PAL

Traditionally, air leaks were defined as prolonged if they persisted longer than 7 days.[6] Current opinion, however, has evolved to consider an air leak as prolonged when it increases length of an otherwise uncomplicated postoperative hospitalization. Accordingly, PAL most recently has been defined as an air leak persisting more than five days (the current median hospital stay of a lobectomy). The databases of the Society of Thoracic Surgeons and European Society of Thoracic Surgeons have both adopted this definition of PAL. To facilitate comparison between different centers and investigations, future studies on air leak should adopt this definition as a reference and perform their analyses accordingly. This would provide consistency in the interpretation and reporting of results and allow for more generalizable comparisons among studies.

## RISK FACTORS

Several studies have attempted to identify risk factors for PAL after pulmonary resection. A recent review has summarized the different risk factors that have been found in the literature.[4] The most

[a] Division of Thoracic Surgery, Umberto I Regional Hospital, Ospedali Riuniti, Ancona 60020, Italy
[b] Division of General Thoracic Surgery, Mayo Clinic, 200 First Street SW, Rochester, MN 55905, USA
* Corresponding author.
E-mail address: brunellialex@gmail.com

Thorac Surg Clin 20 (2010) 359–364
doi:10.1016/j.thorsurg.2010.03.002

consistently reported risk factors are reduced pulmonary function,[6,7,11–13] indicative of a damaged and fragile lung parenchyma, the use of steroids,[14] the performance of an upper lobectomy,[6,13] and presence of pleural adhesions.[6]

The main purpose of this article is, however, to combine these risk factors in models or scores that could be used in the clinical practice or for research purposes to stratify the risk of PAL. Based on their clinical prospective database, the authors used different methods to develop and validate these systems.

## PAL LOGISTIC RISK MODEL
### Objective

The objective of this analysis was to develop a logistic regression equation to predict the risk of an air leak longer than 5 days after pulmonary lobectomy.

### Patients and Methods

An observational analysis was performed on a prospective electronic database. All pulmonary lobectomies operated on at the authors' institution from January 2000 through September 2009 were included. Patients undergoing complex resections including chest wall or diaphragm, or those needing postoperative mechanical ventilation at any time were not included in this series. As a rule, pulmonary lobectomies were performed through a muscle-sparing, nerve-sparing antero-lateral thoracotomy by board-certified general thoracic surgeons. No pleural tents, sealants, buttressing material, or pneumoperitoneum were used in any of these patients. Mechanical staplers were used to close the bronchus in all patients and to complete partially or completely fused fissures in 80% of patients. Twenty percent of patients had complete or filmy fissures that did not require the use of staplers. Systematic lymphadenectomy was performed in all cases at the end of the procedures. At the completion of the operation, the presence of air leak was checked by submerging the lung parenchyma in sterile saline and by reinflating the lung up to a sustained pressure of 25 to 30 cm $H_2O$. If any significant air leak was detected, an attempt was made to eradicate the leak with closure by sutures. Two tubes (until June 2007) or only one chest tube (since July 2007) were positioned in the chest at the completion of the procedure. Chest tubes were left on suction (-15 cm $H_2O$) until the morning after surgery and then managed by using an alternate suction regimen (passive suction or water-seal/gravity mode during the day, active suction during the night, as per institutional protocol).[15]

As a rule all patients were extubated in the operating room and cared for on a specialized thoracic surgical ward. In the rare circumstances in which a patient required intensive care assistance or prolonged mechanical ventilation for major cardiopulmonary complications, the patient was excluded from this analysis to avoid potential confounding factors influencing the duration or assessment of air leak. Thoracotomy chest pain was assessed at least twice during daily rounds and was controlled by using an intravenous continuous infusion of non-opiate drugs titrated to achieve a pain score below 4 (Likert 0 to 10 scale) during the first 72 postoperative hours. Physical rehabilitation and chest physiotherapy were performed in all patients starting on the first postoperative day.

After a chest x-ray was obtained to show satisfactory lung expansion, chest tubes were removed if no air leak was detectable in the chest drain unit and the pleural drainage was less than 400 mL over the preceding 24 hours. When the presence of an air leak was in question, a provocative chest tube clamping was performed for 12 hours. If no symptoms of dyspnea, oxygen desaturation or subcutaneous emphysema ensued, the chest tube was then removed.

### Statistical Analysis

A series of individual risk factors were tested for possible association with PAL greater than 5 days. Variables were initially screened by univariate analysis. Normal distribution of continuous variables was tested by using the Shapiro-Wilk normality test. The numeric variables with a normal distribution were compared by using the unpaired Student's $t$-test. Those with non-normal distribution were tested by using the Mann Whitney test. Categorical variables were compared by using the Chi-square test or Fisher's exact test as appropriate. All variables with $P<.1$ at univariate analysis were used as independent predictors in a stepwise logistic regression analysis (dependent variable: presence of air leak longer than 5 days). To avoid multicollinearity, only one variable in a set of variables with a correlation coefficient greater than 0.5 was selected (by bootstrap) for use in the logistic regression analysis. Bootstrap resampling was used to assess reliability and stability of the significant predictors. Statistical analysis was performed by using Stata 9.0 statistical software. All tests were two-tailed with a significance level of 0.05.

### Results

A total of 777 pulmonary lobectomies were included in the analysis. The mortality rate was

1% (9 patients). Of the 768 patients surviving the operation, 102 had PAL (13%). Univariate analysis showed that the following factors were associated with PAL: forced expiratory volume in the first second of expiration (FEV$_1$) ($P = .002$), FEV$_1$/FVC ratio ($P<.0001$), residual volume to total lung capacity ratio ($P = .08$), carbon monoxide lung diffusion capacity (DLCO) ($P = .001$), smoking pack-years ($P = .08$), presence of pleural adhesions (defined as diffuse dense adhesions involving an entire lobe or more than 30% of the lung surface) ($P<.0001$), use of systemic steroids ($P = .09$).

The authors were not able to find any association between PAL and age, body mass index (BMI), length of stapled parenchyma, right versus left side, location of resected lobe, and induction chemotherapy.

Stepwise logistic regression analysis showed that FEV$_1$ (bootstrap frequency 57%, $P = .008$, odds ratio [OR] 0.98, standard error [SE] 0.97 to 0.99) and presence of adhesions (bootstrap frequency 98%, $P<.0001$, OR 2.42, SE 1.6 to 3.8) were the only significant and reliable predictors independently associated with PAL. The following regression equation estimating the risk of PAL was thus generated:

$\text{Ln } (R/R-1) = -0.8 -0.016 \times \text{FEV}_1 +0.887 \times$ presence of adhesions (Hosmer Lemeshow goodness of fit test 9.9, $P = .3$; c-index 0.66).

## PAL AGGREGATE RISK SCORE
### Objective

Several studies have tested the efficacy of different preventative air leak measures.[16] The interpretation of their results, however, often is complicated by the inclusion of heterogeneous populations and possible selection biases. A system to classify the degree of risk of developing air leak would be desirable in this setting and would make patient selection consistent across different investigators. Thus, the objective of this analysis was to develop a ready-to-use aggregate risk score to stratify the risk of PAL following pulmonary lobectomy.

### Patients and Methods

An observational multicenter analysis was performed using prospective electronic databases. All consecutive pulmonary lobectomies operated on from January 2000 through April 2008 in center A were used as the derivation set to develop the scoring system predicting the risk of PAL greater than 5 days. The risk score was then validated on a sample of patients operated on in another center (center B) from 2006 to 2008. Patients undergoing complex resections including chest

wall or diaphragm, or those needing postoperative mechanical ventilation at any time after the operation were not included in this series. All patients in both centers were operated on by board-certified general thoracic surgeons through a muscle-sparing anterolateral thoracotomy. Mechanical staplers were used to close the bronchus in all patients and to complete partially or completely fused fissures in 80% of patients. Twenty percent of patients had complete or filmy fissures that did not require the use of staplers. No pleural tents, sealants, buttressing material, or pneumoperitoneum were used in any patients. Systematic lymphadenectomy was performed in all cases the end of the operation. At completion of the operation, the presence of an air leak was assessed by submerging the lung parenchyma in sterile saline and by reinflating the lung up to a sustained pressure of 25 to 30 cm $H_2O$. If any significant air leak was detected, an attempt was made to eradicate the leak with closure by sutures. Up to two chest tubes were used to drain the pleural space at the end of the operation. Chest tubes were left on suction (-15/-20 cm $H_2O$) until the morning of the first postoperative day and then managed by using an alternate suction regimen (passive suction during the day, active suction during the night, as per institutional protocol).[15]

In both centers, standardized pathways of care were followed. Patients usually were extubated in the operating room and admitted to a specialized dedicated thoracic ward. Postoperative chest pain was assessed at least twice a day during morning and evening rounds. Treatment was titrated to achieve a pain score below 4 (range 0 to 10) during the first 72 postoperative hours by means of epidurals or continuous intravenous infusion of nonopioid analgesics. Physical rehabilitation and chest physiotherapy were performed in all patients starting from on the first postoperative day. Chest tubes were removed if no air leak was detectable in the chest drain unit and the pleural effusion was less than 400 mL in the preceding 24 hours, as long as a chest radiograph demonstrated satisfactory lung expansion.

### Statistical Analysis

The derivation set consisted of 658 consecutive patients who underwent pulmonary lobectomy in center A. This sample was used to develop the risk-adjusted score predicting the incidence of PAL (>5 days). Initially a series of factors was screened by univariate analysis for possible association with PAL. For the purpose of this analysis and to build the aggregate score, significant numeric variables were dichotomized by using receiver operating characteristics (ROC) analysis (identifying the best cut-off). Significant variables at univariate analysis then were used as independent predictors in a stepwise logistic regression analysis (dependent variable: presence of PAL >5 days). The reliability of the predictors finally assessed was by using a bootstrap resampling technique. Only significant and reliable (bootstrap frequency >50% in 1000 simulated samples) predictors were used to construct the aggregate score. The scoring system was developed by proportional weighting of the significant predictors estimates, assigning a value of 1 to the smallest coefficient. The score was generated by summing each factor score in each patient, and patients then were grouped in classes of incremental risk according to their score.

The risk score then was validated on patients operated on in center B (external validation set), and the risk of PAL was verified in each class in this external population. Moreover, to further assess the stability of the score across different external populations, bootstrap was used to generate 1000 simulated external samples drawn with replacement from the center B population. The proportion of patients with PAL then was verified for each class in each of these new samples.

### Results

The incidence of PAL in the derivation set was 13% (87 of 658 cases). After ROC analysis was used to categorize the numeric variables, stepwise logistic regression identified the following significant and reliable predictors of PAL: age greater than 65 years (coefficient 0.558), presence of pleural adhesions (0.616), $FEV_1$ les than 80% of predicted (0.795), and BMI less than 25.5 (1.03). Based on their coefficients, the individual factor scores were the following: age greater than 65, 1 point; presence of adhesions, 1 point; $FEV_1$ less than 80%, 1.5 points; BMI less than 25.5, 2 points. To obtain a cumulative score, the individual points were summed in each patient to obtain a range from 0 to 5.5. As an example, a 70-year-old patient with an $FEV_1$ of 60%, BMI of 23, and with pleural adhesions would have the maximum score of 5.5 points. Patients then were grouped into four risk classes according to their aggregate scores, which were significantly associated with incremental risk of PAL in the validation set of 233 patients (**Tables 1** and **2**).

When the risk classes were assessed in 1000 bootstrapped samples from center B, the authors found that in class A, 37% of samples had a PAL risk less than 1%, and 98% had a risk less than 5%.

**Table 1**
**Examples of estimated risk of PAL based on different combinations of the predictors in the logistic risk model**

| Case | FEV1% | Pleural Adhesions | Risk of PAL |
|------|-------|-------------------|-------------|
| 1 | 80 | No | 11% |
| 2 | 60 | No | 15% |
| 3 | 50 | No | 17% |
| 4 | 40 | No | 19% |
| 5 | 80 | Yes | 23% |
| 6 | 60 | Yes | 29% |
| 7 | 50 | Yes | 33% |
| 8 | 40 | Yes | 37% |

Class B had a risk less than 10% in 99% of samples. On the other hand, class C had a risk greater than 10% in 91% of samples (although in no cases >20%), and class D had a PAL risk greater than 20% in 99% of samples (in 36% of samples >30%).

### DIGITAL PAL RISK SCORE
#### Objective

New digital chest drainage systems quantify air leak flow and intrapleural pressure in real time and throughout the duration of the chest tube drainage. The objective of this prospective observational study was to evaluate the association between the air flow and intrapleural pressures measured during the immediate postoperative period after lobectomy and the risk of PAL.

#### Population

A retrospective analysis was performed on prospectively collected data from 145 consecutive patients undergoing pulmonary lobectomy in two centers. For the purpose of this analysis, patients undergoing lung resection associated with chest wall or diaphragm resections or needing postoperative ventilator assistance were not included.

All patients were operated on by board-certified general thoracic surgeons. Partially complete or fused fissures were completed by means of mechanical staplers. The bronchus was stapled in most cases. As a rule, up to two chest tubes were positioned at the end of the operation. Chest tubes were left on suction (-20 cm $H_2O$) until the morning of the first postoperative day and then managed by using an alternate suction regimen (passive suction during the day, active suction during the night, as per institutional protocol) or passive suction, according to individual institutional policies.[15]

**Table 2**
**Incidence of PAL greater than 5 days in derivation and validation sets**

| PAL Score Class | Derivation Set (658 patients) | Validation Set (233 patients) |
|---|---|---|
| Class A (score 0) | 1.4% | 0 |
| Class B (score 1) | 5% | 6.7% |
| Class C (score 1.5–3) | 12.5% | 10.9% |
| Class D (score > 3) | 29% | 25.7% |
| Chi2, p value | <0.0001 | 0.003 |
| C-index | 0.71 (95% confidence limit [CL] 0.65-0.77) | 0.69 (95% CL 0.59.0.77) |

Measurements of the air flow and maximum and minimum intrapleural pressures were recorded during the sixth postoperative hour (with all patients on active suction) using a Digivent-MEMS technology (Medela, Switzerland) and averaged for the analysis. For the purpose of this study, a PAL was defined as an air leak lasting longer than 72 hours. For the purpose of this investigation, cessation of air leak was defined as an air flow lower than 10 mL/min during 6 consecutive hours.

## Statistical Analysis

Univariate analysis was first used to screen several perioperative factors (age gender, side and site of operation, $FEV_1$, DLCO, air flow at the sixth hour, differential pressure maximum minus minimum intrapleural pressure at the sixth hour) for possible association with PAL. Significant factors then were used as independent predictors in a stepwise logistic regression analysis (dependent variable: presence of PAL), which was in turn validated by bootstrap resampling technique using 1000 samples.

## Results

Twenty-six patients had an air leak lasting longer than 72 hours (18%). The average air leak flow, maximum and minimum pleural pressures at the sixth postoperative hour were 86 mL/min (range: 0 to 1100), -11.4 cm $H_2O$ and -21.9 cm $H_2O$, respectively. Logistic regression showed that the mean air leak flow (regression coefficient 0.003, $P = .007$, bootstrap frequency 82%) and the mean differential pleural pressure (DeltaP: maximum–minimum intrapleural pressure) (regression coefficient 0.05, $P = .02$, bootstrap frequency 67%) measured during the sixth postoperative hour were significant predictors of PAL, independent of age, $FEV_1$, chronic obstructive pulmonary disease [COPD] status, DLCO, and side and site of lobectomy. ROC analysis was used to find the best cut-offs for air leak flow (50 mL/min) and differential pleural pressure (10 cm $H_2O$). The following four combinations of cutoffs obtained by ROC analysis showed incremental risk of PAL: a. DeltaP less than 10+Flow less than 50: 4% (3 of 73) b. DeltaP greater than 10+Flow less than 50: 15% (5 of 33) c. DeltaP less than 10+Flow greater than 50: 36% (5 of 14) d. DeltaP greater than 10+Flow greater than 50: 52% (13 of 25). Of the patients with flow less than 50 mL/min, those who had a DeltaP greater than 10 cmH2O had close to a fourfold higher risk of PAL. For patients with a flow greater than 50 mL/min and a deltaP greater than 10 cm $H_2O$ (group D), the risk of air leak was 13-fold higher than for patients in group A.

## SUMMARY

The authors have tried to develop practical risk models that could be used for clinical and scientific purposes. These scores may be used during the preoperative patients' counseling phase, by providing reliable information about the risk of developing PAL and the possibility of being discharged with a portable chest drainage unit according to institutional fast track policies. Risk models or risk scores also can be used to identify patients at higher risk for PAL who may benefit the most from the use of preventative measures such as the use of sealants, buttressed staple lines, or pleural tents. Furthermore, they may assist in standardizing inclusion criteria for future randomized clinical trials testing the efficacy of these new technologies, and in doing so make the interpretation of results across different centers and studies more comparable. The clinical use of digital chest drainage units that permit quantitative measurement and recording of air leak flow and intrapleural pressure appears to add to the prediction and management of air leak after pulmonary resection. The use of risk scores based on these digital measures may set the stage for future investigations of active pleural management aimed at treating air leak by tailoring the level of intrapleural pressure to the needs of individual patients.

## REFERENCES

1. Okereke I, Murthy SC, Alster JM, et al. Characterization and importance of air leak after lobectomy. Ann Thorac Surg 2005;79(4):1167–73.
2. Antanavicius G, Lamb J, Papasavas P, et al. Initial chest tube management after pulmonary resection. Am Surg 2005;71(5):416–9.
3. Cerfolio RJ, Tummala RP, Holman WL, et al. A prospective algorithm for the management of air leaks after pulmonary resection. Ann Thorac Surg 1998;66(5):1726–31.
4. Singhal S, Ferraris VA, Bridges CR, et al. Management of alveolar air leak following pulmonary resection. Ann Thorac Surg 2010;89:1327–35.
5. Cerfolio RJ, Bass CS, Pask AH, et al. Predictors and treatment of persistent air leaks. Ann Thorac Surg 2002;73(6):1727–30 [discussion: 1730–1].
6. Brunelli A, Monteverde M, Borri A, et al. Predictors of prolonged air leak after pulmonary lobectomy. Ann Thorac Surg 2004;77(4):1205–10 [discussion: 1210].
7. Bardell T, Petsikas D. What keeps postpulmonary resection patients in hospital? Can Respir J 2003; 10(2):86–9.
8. Irshad K, Feldman LS, Chu VF, et al. Causes of increased length of hospitalization on a general thoracic surgery service: a prospective observational study. Can J Surg 2002;45(4):264–8.
9. Varela G, Jimenez MF, Novoa N, et al. Estimating hospital costs attributable to prolonged air leak in pulmonary lobectomy. Eur J Cardiothorac Surg 2005;27(2):329–33.
10. Brunelli A, Xiume F, Al Refai M, et al. Air leaks after lobectomy increase the risk of empyema but not of cardiopulmonary complications: a case-matched analysis. Chest 2006;130(4):1150–6.
11. Linden PA, Bueno R, Colson YL, et al. Lung resection in patients with preoperative FEV1 < 35% predicted. Chest 2005;127(6):1984–90.
12. Stolz AJ, Schutzner J, Lischke R, et al. Predictors of prolonged air leak following pulmonary lobectomy. Eur J Cardiothorac Surg 2005;27(2):334–6.
13. Abolhoda A, Liu D, Brooks A, et al. Prolonged air leak following radical upper lobectomy: an analysis of incidence and possible risk factors. Chest 1998; 113(6):1507–10.
14. Cerfolio RJ. Chest tube management after pulmonary resection. Chest Surg Clin N Am 2002;12(3): 507–27.
15. Brunelli A, Sabbatini A, Xiume F, et al. Alternate suction reduces prolonged air leak after pulmonary lobectomy: a randomized comparison versus water seal. Ann Thorac Surg 2005;80(3):1052–5.
16. Brunelli A, Varela G, Refai M, et al. A scoring system to predict the risk of prolonged air leak after lobectomy. Ann Thorac Surg 2010, in press.

# Surgical Techniques to Avoid Parenchymal Injury During Lung Resection (Fissureless Lobectomy)

Keki R. Balsara, MD[a], S. Scott Balderson, PA-C[a],
Thomas A. D'Amico, MD[b],*

**KEYWORDS**

- Thoracoscopic surgery • Lobectomy
- Minimally invasive surgery • Outcomes
- Surgical complications

Video-assisted thoracic surgery (VATS), also called thoracoscopic surgery, refers to minimally invasive chest surgery that avoids rib spreading and rib resection and relies entirely on cameras and video technology for visualization. Although popularized in the last decade, it traces its roots back to the early part of the last century when the use of a cystoscope to lyse adhesions in the treatment of tuberculosis was described.[1]

With the advent of laparoscopic surgery for many complicated abdominal procedures, the use of similar technology for thoracic procedures gained popularity. Evidence suggests that thoracoscopic lobectomy can be performed with similar, if not reduced, morbidity and equivalent oncologic outcomes compared with open lobectomy.[2–5] Despite the potential advantages of minimally invasive surgery, only 20% of pulmonary resections are completed using the thoracoscopic technique at present.[6] There are still several potential barriers to adoption of thoracoscopic lobectomy. The belief that pulmonary artery bleeding would be uncontrollable thoracoscopically is an obstacle that is likely to dissuade surgeons from considering learning thoracoscopic lobectomy. Most practicing thoracic surgeons in Europe and North America completed their training before the advent of thoracoscopic lobectomy, and postgraduate training is an extensive process. It is probable that most training programs in thoracic surgery provide exposure to thoracoscopic lobectomy, but the actual operative experience of residents and fellows is unknown.

Recently, single and multi-institutional studies have shown thoracoscopic lobectomy to be an accepted oncologic procedure for patients with early stage lung cancer.[2–5] Thoracoscopic lobectomy has been shown to decrease morbidity, including shorter length of stay, shorter chest tube duration, decreased postoperative pain, improved preservation of pulmonary function, reduced inflammatory response, and shorter recovery time, compared with conventional thoracotomy.[6–9] In addition, it has been shown that thoracoscopic lobectomy is safer than lobectomy by thoracotomy, because it is associated with fewer postoperative complications.[3,4,10]

The indications for thoracoscopic lobectomy are similar to those for lobectomy using an open approach. Absolute contraindications to

Conflict of Interest: None.

[a] Department of Surgery, Duke University Medical Center, Durham, NC 27710, USA

[b] Department of Surgery, Duke University Medical Center, Box 3496, Duke South, White Zone, Room 3589, Durham, NC 27710, USA

* Corresponding author.

E-mail address: damic001@mc.duke.edu

Thorac Surg Clin 20 (2010) 365–369

doi:10.1016/j.thorsurg.2010.04.002

thoracoscopic lobectomy include inability to achieve complete resection with lobectomy, active N2 or N3 disease, and inability to maintain single lung ventilation. Relative contraindications include tumor size, which may preclude a minimally invasive approach to extraction, previous thoracic irradiation and previous thoracotomy.

Several surgical strategies have been used to perform an anatomic lobectomy using a variety of incisions to facilitate dissection. The authors believe that the method described in the following sections provides equivalent oncologic results and minimizes peri- and postoperative complications.

## BASIC PRINCIPLES

Single lung ventilation is required and may be achieved with a dual-lumen endotracheal tube or a bronchial blocker. The patient is placed in the lateral decubitus position. It is helpful to limit the tidal volume to increase the space within the thorax. Most thoracoscopic lobectomies may be performed via 2 or 3 incisions, and the overwhelming majority in the authors' experience have been performed with only 2 incisions.

In general, the port positions are the same whether an upper, lower, or middle lobectomy is performed. The first port, placed in the seventh innerspace in the midaxillary line, is used predominantly for camera placement and, ultimately, chest tube placement. The second port is placed in the fifth or sixth intercostal space in the anterior axillary line. This site is chosen, in part, to allow easy access to hilar structures and to allow for extraction of the specimen (**Fig. 1**).

Perhaps the greatest adjustment for a surgeon transitioning from open lobectomy to thoracoscopic lobectomy is the sequence of dissection required to minimize air leaks. Whereas most surgeons perform open lobectomy using dissection through the fissures, thoracoscopic lobectomy is usually performed by addressing the hilar structures first, and by completing the fissure with a stapling device last.[11] The avoidance of surgical dissection in the fissure is believed to minimize the risk of air leaks.[2]

Instrumentation is critically important when performing thoracoscopic surgery. This procedure requires a 30° videoscope and long, curved instruments to allow for ease of retraction and dissection. High-definition video equipment improves visualization for difficult dissections. Linear staplers are used to control and divide lung parenchyma, vessels, and bronchus (**Fig. 2**).

Once access to the chest has been achieved, thoracoscopic examination is undertaken. The lung parenchyma is assessed for the presence of a mass, additional disease, metastatic disease, and adhesions. For each anatomic lobectomy (described in detail in the following sections), the specific pulmonary vein is the first structure to be divided. Another advantage of the hilar dissection technique is minimization of back and forth retraction; dissection for an upper lobe, for example, begins anteriorly and progresses in the posterior direction only. Most of the hilar dissection may be performed bluntly, with either a dissecting instrument or a thoracoscopic suction device, which also keeps the field dry during dissection. At the conclusion of the dissection, the fissure is completed with the stapling device and the specimen is removed using a protective bag. Mediastinal lymphadenectomy is subsequently performed, although this may be done before hilar dissection at the surgeon's discretion.

In addition to the dissection strategy, which varies according to the lobe being resected, the surgeon should have a planned strategy for conversion if bleeding is encountered or if there is failure to progress with the dissection thoracoscopically. Most of

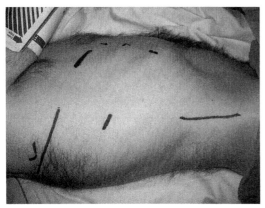

**Fig. 1.** Port placement.

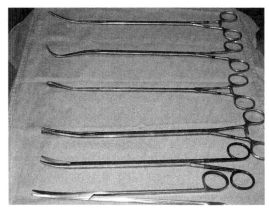

**Fig. 2.** Instruments.

the bleeding encountered can be controlled with direct pressure using a sponge stick; conversion need not be performed emergently.

## RIGHT UPPER LOBECTOMY

Once the right side of the chest has been entered, the lung is retracted medially and dissection along the posterior pleura is performed at the level of the bronchial bifurcation, which facilitates bronchial dissection later from the anterior approach. The lung is then reflected posteriorly and the pulmonary veins are identified. Dissection is performed to identify the bifurcation of the upper and middle lobe veins. Once the upper lobe vein has been clearly identified, it is circumferentially dissected free and divided with a vascular stapler. This procedure reveals the underlying pulmonary artery. In a similar manner, the pulmonary arteries to the upper lobe are mobilized and divided, beginning with the truncus anterior (**Fig. 3**). The last structure to be dissected is usually the bronchus; however, occasionally the bronchus is divided before dissection of the posterior ascending artery. After dividing the bronchus, the fissures are developed and divided using stapling devices, and the specimen is extracted from the chest in a protective bag.[11]

## LEFT UPPER LOBECTOMY

Thoracoscopic left upper lobectomy is performed in a manner similar to that performed on the right side.[11] Posterior dissection is undertaken first to divide the pleural reflection and to identify the posterior artery; as with the right upper lobe, this posterior dissection greatly facilitates the completion from the anterior approach. With the lung retracted posteriorly, dissection is used to identify both pulmonary veins (to ascertain that a common pulmonary vein is not present). The superior pulmonary vein is then encircled and divided, revealing the underlying pulmonary artery and upper lobe bronchus (**Fig. 4**). Dissection of the lymph nodes between the cephalad aspect of the bronchus and the arterial trunk (to the anterior and apical segments) facilitates the ultimate arterial dissection. The branches of the arterial trunk can now be individually exposed and divided, followed by division of the posterior branch. Bronchial dissection and division is now easily accomplished, and is followed by division of the lingular artery. The major fissure is divided with the stapling device (**Fig. 5**).

## LEFT AND RIGHT LOWER LOBECTOMY

There are 2 basic strategies for lower lobectomy, both of which begin with division of the inferior pulmonary ligament, followed by dissection and division of the inferior pulmonary vein. The preferred method does not involve dissection within the fissure (which is stapled last, as with upper lobectomy).[11] After dividing the vein, attention is directed to the bronchus by retracting the lobe cranially, a perspective not obtained via thoracotomy. A plane is created between the bronchus and the artery by dissecting close to the bronchus, which is then divided. For right lower lobectomy, this dissection is begun at the bifurcation with the middle lobe bronchus, which must be preserved. The arterial trunk is then encircled and divided, although it is sometimes easier to divide the branches to the superior and basilar segments individually. Ultimately, the fissure is divided, and the specimen removed.

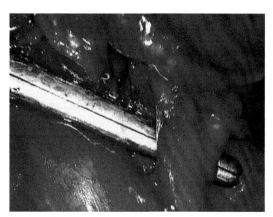

**Fig. 3.** Hilar anatomy of the upper lobe of the right lung.

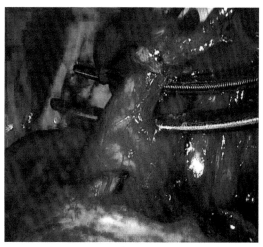

**Fig. 4.** Hilar anatomy of the upper lobe of the left lung.

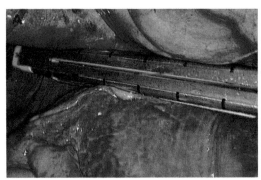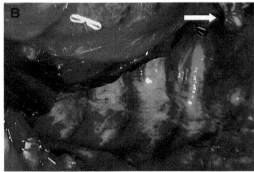

**Fig. 5.** Completion of the horizontal and oblique fissures with the stapler. (*A*) The stapler is engaged across the horizontal fissure. (*B*) By retracting the lung by the bronchial stump (*arrow*), the completion of the fissure is optimized at the hilar level.

## ADVANCED TECHNIQUES

As comfort and facility with thoracoscopic lobectomy increases, it is being more readily applied to more complex cases and surgical interventions, including sleeve lobectomy[12] and segmentectomy.[13–15] Although there have been no studies demonstrating the advantages of these thoracoscopic techniques compared with the conventional procedures, it is probable that the avoidance of rib spreading and the use of modern thoracoscopic techniques confers similar advantages, such as less pain, fewer air leaks, shorter length of stay, and a lower rate of complications.

## OUTCOMES

Using a prospective database, the outcomes of patients who underwent lobectomy at Duke University Medical Center from 1999 to 2009 were analyzed with respect to postoperative complications.[3] Propensity-matched groups were analyzed, based on preoperative variables and stage. Of the 1079 patients in the study, 697 underwent thoracoscopic lobectomy and 382 underwent lobectomy by thoracotomy. In the overall analysis, thoracoscopic lobectomy was associated with a lower incidence of prolonged air leak ($P$ = .0004), atrial fibrillation ($P$ = .01), atelectasis ($P$ = .0001), transfusion ($P$ = .0001), pneumonia ($P$ = .001), sepsis ($P$ = .008), renal failure ($P$ = .003), and death ($P$ = .003). In the propensity-matched analysis based on preoperative variables, comparing 284 patients in each group, 196 patients (69%) who underwent thoracoscopic lobectomy had no complications compared with 144 patients (51%) who underwent thoracotomy ($P$ = .0001). In addition, thoracoscopic lobectomy was associated with fewer prolonged air leaks

(13% vs 19%; $P$ = .05), a lower incidence of atrial fibrillation (13% vs 21%; $P$ = .01), less atelectasis (5% vs 12%; $P$ = .006), fewer transfusions (4% vs 13%; $P$ = .002), less pneumonia (5% vs 10%; $P$ = .05), less renal failure (1.4% vs 5%; $P$ = .02), shorter chest tube duration (median 3 vs 4 days; $P$<.0001), and shorter length of hospital stay (median 4 vs 5 days; $P$<.0001).[3]

Similar results were obtained when the Society of Thoracic Surgeons (STS) database was analyzed by Paul and colleagues.[4] All patients undergoing lobectomy as the primary procedure via thoracoscopy or thoracotomy from 2002 to 2007 were identified in the STS database. After exclusions, 6323 patients were identified: 5042 underwent thoracotomy, 1281 thoracoscopy. A propensity analysis was performed, incorporating preoperative variables, and the incidence of postoperative complications was compared. Matching based on propensity scores produced 1281 patients in each group for analysis of postoperative outcomes. After VATS lobectomy, 945 patients (73.8%) had no complications, compared with 847 patients (65.3%) who had lobectomy via thoracotomy ($P$<.0001). Compared with open lobectomy, VATS lobectomy was associated with a lower incidence of arrhythmias (n = 93 [7.3%] vs n = 147 [11.5%]; $P$ = .0004), reintubation (n = 18 [1.4%] vs n = 40 [3.1%]; $P$ = .0046), and blood transfusion (n = 31 [2.4%] vs n = 60 [4.7%]; $P$ = .0028), as well as a shorter length of stay (4.0 vs 6.0 days; $P$<.0001) and shorter chest tube duration (3.0 vs 4.0 days; $P$<.0001). There was no difference in operative mortality between the 2 groups.[4]

Berry and colleagues[16] reported a recent analysis of high-risk patients aged older than 70 years. During the study period, 338 patients older than 70 years (mean age 75.7±0.2 years) underwent lobectomy (219 thoracoscopy, 119 thoracotomy). Operative mortality was 3.8% (13 patients) and morbidity was 47% (159 patients). Patients with at least 1 complication had increased length of stay (8.3 ± 0.6 vs 3.8 ± 0.1 days; $P<.0001$) and mortality (6.9% [11 of 159] vs 1.1% [2 of 179]; $P = .008$). Significant predictors of morbidity by multivariable analysis included age (odds ratio 1.09; $P = .01$) and thoracotomy as surgical approach (odds ratio 2.21; $P = .004$). Thoracotomy remained a significant predictor of morbidity when the propensity to undergo thoracoscopy was considered (odds ratio 4.9; $P = .002$).[16]

## FISSURELESS LOBECTOMY BY THORACOTOMY

The hilar technique to achieve lobectomy is not limited to the use of minimally invasive surgery, and this strategy may limit air leaks when performed in thoracotomy as well.[17,18] A recent study, comparing the hilar dissection technique to the more traditional transfissure dissection technique demonstrated that the incidence of postoperative air leak and the length of hospital stay were higher with the traditional approach.[17]

## SUMMARY

Thoracoscopic lobectomy has become an accepted, safe, and oncologically sound procedure compared with open lobectomy. Several studies have reported that it reduces the length of stay, postoperative pain, and postoperative complications, including air leaks. Although there are specific technical considerations that must be taken into account, it is increasingly becoming the preferred method of anatomic lobectomy. Surgeons should be encouraged to embrace the minimally invasive strategy, which may be learned in courses using novel simulation techniques.[19] Future directions suggest that this technique will be expanded to address even the most challenging thoracic procedures.

## REFERENCES

1. Berry MF, D'Amico TA. Complications of thoracoscopic pulmonary resection. Semin Thorac Cardiovasc Surg 2007;19:350–4.
2. Onaitis MW, Petersen PR, Balderson SS, et al. Thoracoscopic lobectomy is a safe and versatile procedure: experience with 500 consecutive patients. Ann Surg 2006;244:420–5.
3. Villamizar NR, Darrabie MD, Burfeind WR, et al. Thoracoscopic lobectomy is associated with lower morbidity compared to thoracotomy. J Thorac Cardiovasc Surg 2009;138:419–25.
4. Paul S, Altorki NK, Sheng S, et al. Thoracoscopic lobectomy is associated with lower morbidity than open lobectomy: a propensity-matched analysis from the STS Database. J Thorac Cardiovasc Surg 2010;139:366–78.
5. D'Amico TA. Long-term outcomes of thoracoscopic lobectomy. Thorac Surg Clin 2008;18:259–62.
6. Boffa DJ, Allen MS, Grab JD, et al. Data from The Society of Thoracic Surgeons General Thoracic Surgery Database: the surgical management of primary lung tumors. J Thorac Cardiovasc Surg 2008;135(2):247–54.
7. Nagahiro I, Andou A, Aoe M, et al. Pulmonary function, postoperative pain, and serum cytokine level after lobectomy: a comparison of VATS and conventional procedure. Ann Thorac Surg 2001;72:362–5.
8. Demmy TL, Curtis JJ. Minimally invasive lobectomy directed toward frail and high-risk patients: a case-control study. Ann Thorac Surg 1999;68(1):194–200.
9. Petersen RP, Pham D, Toloza EM, et al. Thoracoscopic lobectomy: a safe and effective strategy for patients receiving induction therapy for non-small cell lung cancer. Ann Thorac Surg 2006;82(1):214–8 [discussion: 219].
10. Hoksch B, Ablassmaier B, Walter M, et al. [Complication rate after thoracoscopic and conventional lobectomy]. Zentralbl Chir 2003;128(2):106–10 [in German].
11. Burfeind WR, D'Amico TA. Thoracoscopic lobectomy. Operat Tech Thorac Cardiovasc Surg 2004; 9:98–114.
12. Mahtabifard A, Fuller CB, McKenna RJ Jr. Video-assisted thoracic surgery sleeve lobectomy: a case series. Ann Thorac Surg 2008;85(2):S729–32.
13. Atkins BZ, Harpole DH Jr, Mangum JH, et al. Pulmonary segmentectomy by thoracotomy or thoracoscopy: reduced hospital length of stay with a minimally-invasive approach. Ann Thorac Surg 2007;84(4):1107–12 [discussion: 1112–3].
14. D'Amico TA. Thoracoscopic segmentectomy: technical considerations and outcomes. Ann Thorac Surg 2008;85(2):S716–718.
15. Pham D, D'Amico TA. Thoracoscopic segmentectomy. Operat Tech Thorac Cardiovasc Surg 2008; 13:188–203.
16. Berry MF, Hanna J, Tong BC, et al. Risk factors for morbidity after lobectomy for lung cancer in elderly patients. Ann Thorac Surg 2009;88:1093–9.
17. Gomez-Caro A, Roca MJ, Lanzas JR, et al. The approach of fused fissures with fissureless technique decreases the incidence of persistent air leaks after lobectomy. Eur J Cardiothorac Surg 2007;31:203–8.
18. Ng T, Ryder BA, Machan JT, et al. Decreasing the incidence of prolonged air leak after right upper lobectomy with the anterior fissureless technique. J Thorac Cardiovasc Surg 2010;139:1007–11.
19. Meyerson SL, LoCascio F, Balderson SS, et al. An inexpensive, reproducible tissue simulator for teaching thoracoscopic lobectomy. Ann Thorac Surg 2010;89:594–7.

# Intraoperative Measures for Preventing Residual Air Spaces

Gaetano Rocco, MD, FRCS (Ed)*

**KEYWORDS**

- Air leaks • Pleural tent • Pneumoperitoneum
- Muscle flap transposition • Thoracoplasty

*If the hill will not come to Mahomet [Mohammed], Mahomet will go to the hill.*
Francis Bacon (1561–1626)
*Essays, Of Boldness*[1]

Residual space after subtotal pulmonary resection is an underestimated complication that at times can lead to a cascade of untoward events, difficult postoperative scenarios, and major morbidity. Conversely, in a significant proportion of patients, persistent air spaces may not be of functional detriment, representing only a disturbing radiological finding. In these circumstances, close observation of the clinical picture is suggested, summarized in the old adage: "We treat patients, not chest x-rays." Our current knowledge is derived directly from the lessons learned from the surgical management of tuberculosis (see Further reading suggestions). The used and at times abused sentence, "We stand on the shoulders of giants," has never been so true as when dealing with residual spaces.

A major factor in determining residual spaces is the degree of awareness and the versatility of the surgeon in preventing air leaks, usually a direct function of the experience and expertise obtained from years of clinical practice.[2] Two determinants of a residual space can be identified according to the presence of an active air escape from the parenchymal surface or from reduced lung compliance that may impair postoperative reexpansion. In the former situation, intrapleural pressure becomes increasingly positive and the degree of lung collapse strictly depends on the completeness of air evacuation through the drainage system. When loss of parenchymal elastic recoil is the predominant factor causing incomplete reexpansion of the lung, the intrapleural pressure remains stagnant and the application of suction may only induce a temporary volume gain with no functional benefit. Postoperative residual spaces often result from a combination of active air leakage and reduced lung compliance appearing simultaneously or sequentially and contributing to incomplete lung reexpansion. According to the principles mentioned earlier, the surgeon should be aware of three potential types of residual spaces:

1. Physiologic residual space, by definition limited in size and duration, occurs after closure of the chest cavity when air at atmospheric pressure remains trapped in the pleural space. In the presence of adequate lung compliance, the evacuation of this residual air pocket depends primarily on the efficacy of chest drainage in the presence of an airtight chest wound closure.
2. Residual space caused by persistent, active air leakage, which maintains a positive intrapleural pressure by continuous escape of air from the lung (ie, stapled fissures, parenchymal tears, or neglected blebs) thereby leading to its partial collapse.
3. Residual space caused by deficient lung compliance because of age and underlying lung or pleural conditions. This is often the case with pulmonary resections for postprimary tuberculosis, complex

Division of Thoracic Surgery, Department of Thoracic Surgery and Oncology, National Cancer Institute, Pascale Foundation, Naples, Italy
* Via Semmola 81, 80131 Naples, Italy.
E-mail address: Gaetano.Rocco@btopenworld.com

Thorac Surg Clin 20 (2010) 371–375
doi:10.1016/j.thorsurg.2010.03.003
1547-4127/10/$ – see front matter © 2010 Elsevier Inc. All rights reserved.

mycetomas, and bronchiectases. Fibrotic interstitial changes may also lead to restrictive damage. Concomitant pleural infections may induce a significant thickening of the visceral pleura with the attendant entrapment of the lung.

Preventive intraoperative measures tend to address all three potential causes of residual spaces, which can develop alone or in combination. The need for a meticulous surgical technique associated with a carefully devised lung resection strategy, resorting to sealants and chest drain management, are addressed in detail by D'Amico T and Rice TW elsewhere in this issue. The management of the often catastrophic clinical scenario resulting from the presence of a bronchopleural fistula on the main stem or lobar bronchial stump is beyond the scope of this article. The current discussion revolves around intraoperative measures that to obliterate space by reducing the volume of the chest cavity through geometric remodeling of the anatomic boundaries of the lung (**Table 1**).

## THE PARIETAL PLEURA

The creation of a pleural tent to compartmentalize the chest cavity by reducing the volume of apex of the chest, facilitating lung reexpansion after upper lobectomies or lung volume reduction surgery, is a well-known technique that rightfully belongs to the routine thoracic surgical armamentarium.[1,3,4] Brunelli and colleagues[5] have confirmed the usefulness of this procedure in a prospective randomized study on 200 patients subjected to upper lobectomy. The addition of

a pleural tent yielded a reduction in the duration of air leaks by postoperative day 4 and in the overall length of stay.[5] The fundamentals of this technique date back to the late 1950s, when several investigators such as Drewer, Hansen, and Miscal independently conceived the idea of a pleural partition through an apical parietal pleurolysis to avoid lung over expansion following resection for tuberculosis.[1] In brief, the detachment of the parietal pleura from the endothoracic fascia begins at the level of the thoracotomy. Pleural elevation is taken circumferentially along the inner surface of the uppermost chest wall paying attention to avoid tearing the pleura. Careful dissection is needed in the proximity of the thoracic inlet, especially along the costovertebral recess to avoid inadvertent injury to the stellate ganglion. Anteriorly, awareness of the internal mammary bundle is crucial for defining the extension of the dissection. When a thoracoscopic pleural tent is performed,[6] the magnification of the surgical field and the use of an endoscopic swab facilitates this maneuver. The creation of the pleural tent is completed by anchoring the parietal flap to the elevated intercostal muscle with sutures at the thoracotomy wound site. During video-assisted thoracoscopic surgery procedures, clipping of the pleural edges to the inferiorly located ports is meant to attain the same result as in open surgery. The tent compartmentalizes the chest cavity by obliquely separating a caudally located, fully drained sector of the lung from an uppermost smaller empty space, which is allowed to fill with serum, giving the remaining lung enough time to expand. The radiological outcome is represented by a thin apical dense layer representing the fibrotic

**Table 1**
**Possible options to intraoperatively manage residual air spaces (see text)**

| Anatomic Structure | Intraoperative Procedure | Indications |
|---|---|---|
| Parietal pleura | Pleural tent | Upper lobectomies<br>Upper bilobectomy |
| | Pleurectomy, mechanical abrasion, talc | All lobectomies/bilobectomies |
| Visceral pleura | Adhesiolysis | All lobectomies/bilobectomies |
| | Decortication | All lobectomies/bilobectomies |
| Chest wall muscles | Intrathoracic transposition Muscle tent | All lobectomies/bilobectomies |
| Diaphragm | Phrenic nerve paralysis | All lobectomies/bilobectomies |
| | Pneumoperitoneum | Lower lobectomies/lower bilobectomy |
| | Resuspension | Lower lobectomies/lower bilobectomies |
| Osteotendinous chest wall | Rib resection at thoracotomy level | All lobectomies/bilobectomies |
| | Tailored thoracoplasty | Upper lobectomies/bilobectomy |
| Omentum | Flap transposition | All lobectomies/bilobectomies |

regression of the extrapleural collection on the background of a fully expanded lung.[7]

A pleural tent cannot be constructed when the parietal pleura is too thin, obviously diseased, or already dissected; its value in resections other than upper lobectomies/bilobectomies is questionable. In these cases, and in ventilated patients requiring open lung biopsy or on long-term steroids, talc insufflation or mechanical abrasion of the parietal pleura can facilitate pleurodesis.[8]

## THE VISCERAL PLEURA

Primary or secondary (ie, postobstructive pneumonia) chronic inflammatory processes of the lung and pleura may lead to lung trapping. As a consequence, postresectional reexpansion of the residual parenchyma is severely hindered and lung decortication becomes imperative. The removal of the peel from the underlying parenchyma needs to be performed with care to avoid air leaking from unwarranted tears. Collaboration with the anesthesiologist and meticulous surgical technique are of paramount importance to facilitate division of strands of pleural scarring.

## CHEST WALL MUSCLES

Intrathoracic transposition of muscle flaps can respond to two objectives. First, the need to obliterate otherwise empty spaces in any position inside the chest cavity.[9,10] Second, similar to the pleural tent, chest wall muscles can be used to create partitions of the pleural space (muscle tent).[11] One basic technical tenet of muscle flap intrathoracic transfer resides in the preresectional elevation of the muscles, emphasizing the need for careful preoperative planning and a muscle-sparing surgical approach.[9,10] Appropriate knowledge of the vascular supply, conformation, intrathoracic reach, and flap elevation techniques is of paramount importance to devise intraoperative solutions to potential space problems.[9] Intercostal muscles are readily available, but unless elevated from two adjacent spaces, they cannot provide enough bulk to obliterate pleural recesses. Their use can be envisaged to reinforce suture lines, usually bronchial, but also stapled fissures at risk of breakdown (ie, after tuberculosis resections). Traditionally, serratus anterior muscle flaps have been used extensively to cover postresectional bronchial stumps with limited morbidity at the donor site.[12] Albeit providing different muscle bulk, serratus anterior and latissimus dorsi flaps can be transferred together or separately in the chest, especially in the setting of complex infected spaces.[13] The harvesting technique is straightforward inasmuch as the thoracodorsal pedicle is preserved[13] and both muscles can be transposed through a window obtained in the chest wall by a limited resection of a 5- to 6-cm segment of the second rib.[11,13] The choice of this entrance site for muscle transfer is dictated by the need to avoid jeopardizing its blood supply.[11] Once inside the chest, the muscles are loosely anchored to the residual pleura, the periosteum, or the intercostal muscles to allow for gradual lung reexpansion (drawbridge effect).[11] As a consequence, the chest cavity is divided by the muscles into two potentially separate chambers; the uppermost, not vented, is left to fill with serum or to adhere to the apical chest wall. The lowermost chamber is drained and the residual lung is covered by viable muscle bulk conveying oxygen, and if needed, antibiotics.[11]

## THE DIAPHRAGM

In the heroic times of nonresectional treatment, collapse therapy for tuberculous cavitations was a life-saving procedure for patients with complex postprimary sequelae. The concept of inducing an iatrogenic cranial dislocation of the hemidiaphragm by either interrupting or simply crushing the ipsilateral phrenic nerve in its course at the thoracic inlet to facilitate collapse of pulmonary cavitations was introduced in the 1930s.[14] Surprisingly, many contemporary thoracic surgeons have inherited this time-honored approach to the residual space after lung resection despite the potential complications of a sudden and permanent elevation of the diaphragm. Contralateral mediastinal shift with the attendant cardiovascular derangements and abdominal visceral space rearrangement may be responsible for symptoms of different severity. In theory, these side effects are attenuated if the phrenic nerve injury becomes somehow reversible.[15] To this purpose, the phrenic nerve is usually injected with local anesthetic either as single administration or by continuous infusion to ensure the desired volumetric effect.[15–17] In addition, the use of type A botulinum toxin has also been advocated.[18] Reportedly, the standard technique of inducing a transient phrenic nerve paralysis includes identification of the phrenic nerve at the hilum with gentle grasping, avoiding nerve crushing.[15] The local anesthetic (1–2 mL of bupivacaine without epinephrine) is then injected in the proximity of the nerve but into the pericardium.[8,15]

Following the same concept of diaphragmatic dislocation, the pneumoperitoneum has been reported to address the issue of potential residual spaces, irrespective of the type of lobectomy performed.[19] Usually, between 800 and 1000 mL of air is injected transdiaphragmatically after lower lobe resections either as a single instillation or on-demand delivery through a properly positioned catheter according to the appearance on a chest radiograph.[20] The latter method avoids repeated transabdominal injections if the first instillation delivered at thoracotomy is not sufficient. In two prospective studies,[21,22] perioperatively administered pneumoperitoneum was shown to reduce the duration of air leakage and attendant chest drain time. Recently, based on a series of 60 patients randomly assigned to prophylactic pneumoperitoneum or no treatment after lobectomy, one group demonstrated that prophylactically induced pneumoperitoneum could yield shortened hospitalizations compared with nontreated patients.[22] This evidence had been suggested years earlier by Cerfolio and colleagues[23] who focused their attention only on the evolution of residual space after bilobectomy, recommending prophylactic pneumoperiotoneum as a routine space-obliterating procedure. In challenging clinical scenarios, resorting to a combination of pleural tenting, phrenic nerve block and pneumoperitoneum to obliterate significant residual spaces may also be indicated. Resuspension of the diaphragm by circumferential division of its costal attachments and subsequent suturing of the more cranial chest wall could be taken into consideration in rare and extreme circumstances (Lyman Brewer maneuver).[1]

## OSTEOTENDINOUS CHEST WALL

Until some time ago and still today in selected patients (ie, reoperation after major previous thoracic procedure), standard posterolateral thoracotomy includes subperiosteal removal of 1 rib to ensure proper intrathoracic exposure. This maneuver also contributes to reduce the volume of the hemithorax, especially in patients with widened intercostal spaces from significant chronic obstructive pulmonary disease. Modern thoracic surgery rarely contemplates tailored thoracoplasty for routine preventative management of residual spaces by collapsing the apical chest wall.[24,25] However, the resurgence of multidrug-resistant, aggressive tuberculosis and its sequelae or other destructive pulmonary infections in immunocompromised patients may mandate the obliteration of an otherwise unmanageable anatomic area (ie, the apex of the chest) when all other intraoperative measures are unavailable.[24,25]

## OMENTUM

The intraoperative prophylactic measures mentioned earlier are usually sufficient to obliterate potentially threatening air spaces. On the other hand, the usefulness of the omentum in solving complex thoracic problems is well known.[26] In selected circumstances, omental flap transposition can actually be a valuable addition to the surgical armamentarium, especially if harvesting is conducted transdiaphragmatically or via a minimally invasive abdominal approach.[27]

## SUMMARY

In thoracic surgery, the intraoperative solution of difficult air space problems relies heavily on the operating surgeon's creativity, versatility, and meticulous surgical technique, as well us profound knowledge of the anatomy and past surgical heritage. The same degree of expertise and experience is needed to simply observe innocent residual spaces without resorting to unnecessary aggressiveness. Management of residual air spaces is an art that conclusively defines the maturity of a thoracic surgeon.

## REFERENCES

1. Robinson LA, Preksto D. Pleural tenting during upper lobectomy decreases chest tube time and total hospitalization days. J Thorac Cardiovasc Surg 1998;115:319–27.
2. Okereke I, Murthy SC, Alster JM, et al. Characterization and importance of air leak after lobectomy. Ann Thorac Surg 2005;79:1167–73.
3. Okur E, Kir A, Halezeroglu S, et al. Pleural tenting following upper lobectomies or bilobectomies of the lung to prevent residual air space and prolonged air leak. Eur J Cardiothorac Surg 2001;20:1012–5.
4. Brunelli A, Al Refai M, Muti M, et al. Pleural tent after upper lobectomy: a prospective randomized study. Ann Thorac Surg 2000;69:1722–4.
5. Brunelli A, Al Refai M, Monteverde M, et al. Pleural tent after upper lobectomy: a randomized study of efficacy and duration of effect. Ann Thorac Surg 2002;74:1958–62.
6. Venuta F, De Giacomo T, Rendina EA, et al. Thoracoscopic pleural tent. Ann Thorac Surg 1998;66:1833–4.
7. Goodman PC, Minagi H, Thomas AN. Radiographic appearances of the chest after pleural space reduction procedures: construction of a pleural tent and phrenoplasty. Am J Roentgenol 1977;129:229–31.
8. Murthy S. Air leak and pleural space management. Thorac Surg Clin 2006;16:261–5.
9. Arnold PG, Pairolero PC. Intrathoracic muscle flap. Ann Surg 1990;221:656–61.
10. Mathes SJ, Nahai F. Clinical application for muscle and musculocutaneous flaps. St. Louis (MO): Mosby; 1982. p. 95–179.
11. Rocco G. Pleural partition with intrathoracic muscle transposition (muscle tent) to manage residual

spaces after subtotal pulmonary resections. Ann Thorac Surg 2004;78:e74–6.

12. Groth SS, Whitson BA, D'Cunha J, et al. Serratus anterior transposition muscle flaps for bronchial coverage: technique and functional outcomes. Ann Thorac Surg 2009;88:2044–6.

13. Widmer MK, Krueger T, Lardinois D, et al. A comparative evaluation of intrathoracic latissimus dorsi and serratus anterior muscle transposition. Eur J Cardiothorac Surg 2000;18:435–9.

14. Campbell AJ. Diaphragmatic paralysis: a critical review of its use as a therapeutic measure in respiratory disease. Proc R Soc Med 1934;27:1555–62.

15. Carboni GL, Vogt A, Küster JR, et al. Reduction of airspace after lung resection through controlled paralysis of the diaphragm. Eur J Cardiothorac Surg 2008;33:272–5.

16. Clavero JM, Cheyre JE, Solovera ME, et al. Transient diaphragmatic paralysis by continuous para-phrenic infusion of bupivacaine: a novel technique for the management of residual spaces. Ann Thorac Surg 2007;83:1216–8.

17. Kaya SO, Atalay H, Erbay HR, et al. Reduction of airspace after lung resection through controlled paralysis of the diaphragm. Eur J Cardiothorac Surg 2008;33:272–5.

18. Kaya SO, Atalay H, Erbay HR, et al. Exploring strategies to prevent post-lobectomy space: transient diaphragmatic paralysis using Botulinum toxin type A (BTX-A). Int Semin Surg Oncol 2005;19(2):21.

19. De Giacomo T, Rendina EA, Venuta F, et al. Pneumoperitoneum for the management of pleural air space problems associated with major pulmonary resections. Ann Thorac Surg 2001;72:1716–9.

20. Puc MM, Podbielski FJ, Conlan AA. A novel technique for creation of adjustable pneumoperitoneum. Ann Thorac Surg 2004;77:1469–71.

21. Toker A, Dilege S, Tanju S, et al. Perioperative pneumoperitoneum after lobectomy-bilobectomy operations for lung cancer: a prospective study. Thorac Cardiovasc Surg 2003;51:93–6.

22. Okur E, Arisoy Y, Baysungur V, et al. Prophylactic intraoperative pneumoperitoneum decreases pleural space problems after lower lobectomy or bilobectomy of the lung. Thorac Cardiovasc Surg 2009;57:160–4.

23. Cerfolio RJ, Holman WL, Katholi CR. Pneumoperitoneum after concomitant resection of the right middle and lower lobes (bilobectomy). Ann Thorac Surg 2000;70:942–6.

24. Daly RC, Pairolero PC, Piehler JM, et al. Pulmonary aspergilloma. J Thorac Cardiovasc Surg 1986;92:981–8.

25. Grima R, Krassas A, Bagan P, et al. Treatment of complicated pulmonary aspergillomas with cavernostomy and muscle flap: interest of concomitant limited thoracoplasty. Eur J Cardiothorac Surg 2009;36:910–3.

26. D'Andrilli A, Ibrahim M, Andreetti C, et al. Transdiaphragmatic harvesting of the omentum through thoracotomy for bronchial stump reinforcement. Ann Thorac Surg 2009;88:212–5.

27. Shrager JB, Wain JC, Wright CD, et al. Omentum is highly effective in the management of complex cardiothoracic surgical problems. J Thorac Cardiovasc Surg 2003;125:526–32.

## FURTHER READINGS

Barker WL. Natural history of residual air spaces after pulmonary resection. Chest Surg Clin N Am 1996;6:585–613.

Barker WL, Langston HT, Naffah P. Postresectional thoracic spaces. Ann Thorac Surg 1966;2:299–310.

Bell JW. Management of the postresection space in tuberculosis. I. Following segmental and wedge resection. J Thorac Surg 1955;29:649–57.

Bell JW. Management of the postresection space in tuberculosis. II. Following lobectomy. J Thorac Surg 1956;31:442–51.

Bell JW. Management of the postresection space in tuberculosis. III. Role of pre- and postresection thoracoplasty. J Thorac Surg 1956;32:580–92.

Brewer LA 3rd, Gazzaniga AB. Phrenoplasty, a new operation for the management of pleural dead space following pulmonary resection. Ann Thorac Surg 1968;6:119–26.

Deschamps C, Pairolero PC, Allen MS, et al. Management of postpneumonectomy empyema and bronchopleural fistula. Chest Surg Clin N Am 1996;6:519–27.

Ellis FH Jr, Clagett OT, Carr DT. Simultaneous pulmonary resection and thoracoplasty in the treatment of pulmonary tuberculosis. Am Rev Tuberc 1952;65:159–67.

Law SW, Jordan GL. Control of the postresectional space with the Marlex roof. Ann Thorac Surg 1967;3:204–10.

Peppas G, Molnar TF, Jeyasingham K, et al. Thoracoplasty in the context of current surgical practice. Ann Thorac Surg 1993;56:903–9.

Silver AW, Espinas EE, Byron FX. The fate of the postresection space. Ann Thorac Surg 1966;2:311–36.

# Use of Sealants and Buttressing Material in Pulmonary Surgery: An Evidence-Based Approach

Thomas W. Rice, MD[a],*, Eugene H. Blackstone, MD[a,b]

## KEYWORDS

• Air leak • Lung volume reduction surgery • Lobectomy

Air leak complicating pulmonary surgery is inevitable.[1,2] Therefore, it is imperative to minimize its occurrence and adverse consequences. Careful handling of the lung and meticulous operative technique are the foundation to meet these goals. However, unlike control of bleeding, homeostatic and physical mechanisms controlling air leakage are primitive or nonexistent. The problem of air leak is increased by the substantial and fluctuating negative pressure gradient across the pleural surface. Intraoperative attempts to control air leaks proactively with sealants or staple-line buttressing are theoretically promising, potentially valuable, but controversial. The contemporary literature is reviewed, and evidence-based grading,[3] which assesses the qualities of recommendations and evidence (**Table 1**), is used to provide recommendations for intraoperative use of these agents to control air leak complicating pulmonary surgery.

## SEALANTS

An ideal lung sealant should bond rapidly to lung tissue in the presence of air, blood, or moisture, be able to withstand inflation pressures of greater than −40 cm $H_2O$, have sufficient flexibility and compliance to permit lung inflation and deflation, absorb without a trace, be nontoxic, and eliminate air leaks.

The cardiac and vascular experience with fibrin sealants for controlling bleeding led to its illogical application as an agent for controlling air leak complicating pulmonary surgery. Next came attempts to develop synthetic sealants for pulmonary surgery. Today, the usual sealant is collagen fleece coated with fibrin. This evolutionary process is proof that the quest for the perfect lung sealant continues.

### Biologic Sealants

#### Fibrin sealant

Fibrin sealant was developed during World War II to stop bleeding from battle injuries. It is a mixture of components involved in the last step of the coagulation cascade. The principal components are fibrin and thrombin. In the presence of calcium, thrombin cleaves fibrinogen to produce fibrin monomers that polymerize to form insoluble fibrin. Fibrin also has a role in stabilization and early healing of wounds. Commercially available products may include factor XIII, which facilitates cross-linking of fibrin; fibronectin, which facilitates fibrin adhesion; and aprotinin, which stabilizes fibrin.

Funded in part by the Daniel and Karen Lee Endowed Chair in Thoracic Surgery (Dr Rice) and the Kenneth Gee and Paula Shaw, PhD, Chair in Heart Research (Dr Blackstone).

[a] Department of Thoracic and Cardiovascular Surgery, Heart and Vascular Institute, Cleveland Clinic, 9500 Euclid Avenue/Desk J4-1, Cleveland, OH 44195, USA
[b] Department of Quantitative Health Sciences, Research Institute, Cleveland Clinic, 9500 Euclid Avenue/Desk JJ-4, Cleveland, OH 44195, USA
* Corresponding author.
E-mail address: ricet@ccf.org

Thorac Surg Clin 20 (2010) 377–389
doi:10.1016/j.thorsurg.2010.03.008
1547-4127/10/$ – see front matter © 2010 Elsevier Inc. All rights reserved.

**Table 1**
**Grading recommendations**

| Grade of Recommendation and Description | Benefit vs Risk and Burdens | Methodological Quality of Supporting Evidence | Implications |
|---|---|---|---|
| 1A. Strong recommendation, high-quality evidence | Benefits clearly outweigh risk and burdens, or vice versa | RCTs without important limitations or overwhelming evidence from observational studies | Strong recommendation, can apply to most patients in most circumstances without reservation |
| 1B. Strong recommendation, moderate-quality evidence | Benefits clearly outweigh risk and burdens, or vice versa | RCTs with important limitations (inconsistent results, methodological flaws, indirect, or imprecise) or exceptionally strong evidence from observational studies | Strong recommendation, can apply to most patients in most circumstances without reservation |
| 1C. Strong recommendation, low-quality or very low-quality evidence | Benefits clearly outweigh risk and burdens, or vice versa | Observational studies or case series | Strong recommendation, but may change when higher-quality evidence becomes available |
| 2A. Weak recommendation, high-quality evidence | Benefits closely balanced with risks and burdens | RCTs without important limitations or overwhelming evidence from observational studies | Weak recommendation, best action may differ depending on circumstances or patients' or societal values |
| 2B. Weak recommendation, moderate-quality evidence | Benefits closely balanced with risks and burden | RCTs with important limitations (inconsistent results, methodological flaws, indirect, or imprecise) or exceptionally strong evidence from observational studies | Weak recommendation, best action may differ depending on circumstances or patients' or societal values |
| 2C. Weak recommendation, low-quality or very low-quality evidence | Uncertainty in the estimates of benefits, risks, and burden; benefits, risk, and burden may be closely balanced | Observational studies or case series | Very weak recommendations; other alternatives may be equally reasonable |

*Abbreviation:* RCT, randomized clinical trial.

*From* Guyatt G, Gutterman D, Baumann MH, et al. Grading strength of recommendations and quality of evidence in clinical guidelines. Chest 2006;129:176; with permission.

## Experimental evidence

In rats, application of fibrin sealant to suture closure of lung incisions permits statistically significantly higher lung inflation pressure.[4] In contrast, in rabbits, no difference has been found in the ventilatory pressure required to produce air leak with application of fibrin sealant applied to suture closure of pulmonary wedge resections.[5] Suture closure was superior to fibrin sealant alone; however, fibrin sealant produced less hemorrhagic pulmonary necrosis than suture or suture and fibrin sealant closures. In dogs, fibrin sealant applied to a standard pleural defect significantly decreased mean air leak in a 90-minute period compared with controls (2.1–0.5 [mean decrease, 81%] vs 1.4–1.1 L/min [mean decrease, 20%], $P<.0001$), although no explanation was given for the larger initial air leak in the fibrin sealant group.[6] At 3 months, pleural adhesions were similar. In pigs, fibrin sealant was superior to albumin in preventing air leak from wedge resection sites at inflation pressures of 20 cm $H_2O$ ($P<.001$), 30 cm $H_2O$ ($P<.001$), and 45 cm $H_2O$ ($P$ value not stated [NS]), and after 10 minutes of airway clamping after application of sealant and before ventilation ($P = .002$).[7]

Method of application may determine the ability of fibrin sealant to control air leak. In dogs, the sealing effect of fibrin glue was unstable for 12 hours after its application.[8] The application technique that allowed the fibrin seal to reach its full strength fastest was rubbing the target area with fibrinogen and then spraying with fibrinogen and thrombin.

## Clinical evidence

**Lung volume reduction surgery** There has been 1 randomized study evaluating fibrin sealant in lung volume reduction surgery (LVRS) (**Table 2**). In a single-institution study of 25 consecutive patients, Moser and colleagues[9] randomized each side of a bilateral LVRS to receive autologous fibrin sealant sprayed along staple lines (treatment) and not (control) (evidence grade 1B). Intraoperative randomization occurred after completion of LVRS on the first side. Air leaks were independently quantified by 2 blinded observers from 0 (none) to 4 (continuous severe) 1.5 to 2 hours after surgery and twice a day until chest tube removal. Mean total air leak scores for the first 48 hours were $4.7 \pm 7.7$ in the treatment group versus $16 \pm 10$ in controls (nonparametric because of skewed distribution, $P<.001$). Air leak occurred in 14 of 24 versus 23 of 24, respectively. Prolonged air leaks (more than 7 days) were less frequent in the treatment group than in the control group (4.5% vs 32%, respectively, $P = .03$) and duration of chest tube drainage shorter ($2.8 \pm 1.9$

vs $5.9 \pm 2.9$ days, respectively, $P<.001$). Difference in hospital stay could not be assessed because each patient served as his or her own control own control.

**Pulmonary resection** There have been 7 randomized studies evaluating fibrin sealant in pulmonary resections (see **Table 2**). In a single-institution study of 28 consecutive patients undergoing lobectomy, Fleisher and colleagues[10] randomized patients to receive fibrin sealant (fibrinogen, factor XIII, fibronectin, aprotinin, plasminogen, thrombin, and calcium) sprayed onto parenchymal staple lines and any cut surface (treatment) and not (control) (evidence grade 2B). Paradoxically, plasminogen was used in this commercial preparation. Although data were skewed, parametric analyses were used. Comparing treatment with control groups, there was no difference in mean air leak duration ($2.3 \pm 3.7$ vs $3.3 \pm 3.3$ days, respectively, $P>.9$), duration of chest tube drainage ($6.0 \pm 4.1$ vs $5.9 \pm 3.9$ days, respectively, $P>.9$), or hospital stay ($9.8 \pm 3.1$ vs $11.5 \pm 3.9$, respectively, $P = .2$).

In a single-institution study of 50 consecutive patients undergoing bilobectomy or less, including decortication, Wurtz and colleagues[11] randomized 25 patients to receive fibrin sealant (fibrin, fibronectin, factor XIII, aprotinin, thrombin, and calcium) applied to the surgical sites (treatment) and 25 patients not (control) (evidence grade 2B). There was no difference in quality of air leak control, volume of chest tube drainage, residual pleural fluid collection, failed lung expansion following chest tube removal, or hospital stay.

In a second study of 50 consecutive patients undergoing bilobectomy or less, including decortication, Wurtz and colleagues[12] randomized 24 patients to receive fibrin sealant (fibrin, fibronectin, factor XIII, aprotinin, aprotinin, plasminogen, thrombin, and calcium) applied to the surgical sites (treatment) and 25 patients not (control) (evidence grade 2B). Paradoxically, plasminogen was used in this preparation. Comparing treatment with control groups, the magnitude of air leak (as measured by loss of vacuum in the closed thorax) was less in the treatment group ($15 \pm 12$ vs $31 \pm 26$ cm $H_2O$, respectively, $P<.05$). However, there was no difference in volume of chest tube drainage, complications, or hospital stay ($9.9 \pm 2.4$ vs $11 \pm 3.9$ days, respectively, $P = $ NS).

In a single-institution study of 114 consecutive patients undergoing pulmonary resections and decortications, Mouritzen and colleagues[13] randomized 55 to receive fibrin sealant (fibrinogen, factor XIII, aprotinin, thrombin, and calcium) sprayed along staple lines and cut lung surfaces and 59 patients not (control) (evidence grade 2C).

**Table 2**
**Fibrin sealants: findings in RCTs**

| Procedure/ First Author | Reduction in Air Leak | | Duration | Reduction in: | | Difference in: | | Evidence Grade |
| | Magnitude | Incidence | | Chest Tube Duration | Hospital Stay | Cost | Complications | |
|---|---|---|---|---|---|---|---|---|
| LVRS | | | | | | | | |
| Moser et al[9] | ↓ | ↓ | ↓ | ↓ | NA | NS | ± | 1B |
| Resection | | | | | | | | |
| Fleisher et al[10] | NS | NR | ± | ± | ± | NS | ± | 2B |
| Wurtz et al[11] | ± | NR | NR | NR | ± | NS | ± | 2B |
| Wurtz et al[12] | ↓ | NR | NR | NR | ± | NS | ± | 2B |
| Mouritzen et al[13] | NS | ↓ | ± | ± | ± | NS | ± | 2C |
| Wong and Goldstraw[14] | NS | NR | ± | ± | ± | NS | ± | 2B |
| Belboul et al[15] | ↓ | ↓ immediate ± any day | NR | ± | ± | NS | ± | 2A |
| Fabian et al[16] | NS | ↓ | ↓ | ↓ | ± | NS | ± | 2B |
| Metastasectomy | | | | | | | | |
| Brega Massone et al[17] | NS | NR | ↓ | ↓ | ↓ | NS | ± | 2C |

*Abbreviations:* ↓, decrease; ±, no difference; NA, not applicable; NR, not reported; NS, not studied.

Pneumonectomy was performed in 51 patients, 24 in the treatment group and 27 in the control group. In an observational subgroup study of those not undergoing pneumonectomy, fibrin sealant improved intraoperative air leak control, with 81% free from air leaks when airway pressure was raised to 30 cm $H_2O$. Comparing treatment with control groups, fibrin sealant reduced occurrence of air leaks (39% vs 66%, respectively, $P<.02$). Duration of air leak and several minor criteria (outcomes) were not different between groups.

In a single-institution study of 66 patients undergoing lobectomy, segmentectomy, or decortication by a single senior surgeon and judged intraoperatively to have a moderate to severe air leak, Wong and Goldstraw[14] randomized equal numbers to receive fibrin sealant (fibrinogen, factor XIII, fibronectin, aprotinin, thrombin, and calcium) sprayed onto to the raw lung surfaces (treatment) and not (control) (evidence grade 2B). Two independent observers, blinding not stated, assessed outcome. Comparing medians between treatment and control groups, duration of air leak (5 [range, 0.1–22] vs 4 [1–16] days, respectively, $P = .8$), duration of chest tube drainage (6 [range, 2–23] days, respectively, $P = .08$), and hospital stay (8 [range, 4–35] vs 9,[5–20] respectively, $P = .6$) were similar, although parametric tests of

these nonparametric data seem to have been performed.

In a single-institution study of 40 consecutive patients undergoing lobectomy by 1 of 4 surgeons, Belboul and colleagues[15] randomized equal numbers to receive autologous fibrin sealant sprayed onto all dissected areas at risk for air leak and not (control) (evidence grade 2A). A blinded observer made all postoperative assessments. Comparing treatment with control groups, fibrin sealant reduced mean volume of air leak (15 ± 0.3 vs 0.7 ± 0.6 L, respectively, method of measurement not stated, $P = .01$) and occurrence of air leak immediately postoperatively (20% vs 60%, respectively, variability not stated, $P = .02$) but not postoperatively (40% vs 65%, respectively, variability not stated, $P = .2$). There were no differences (median [quartiles]) between the treatment and control groups in duration of chest tube drainage (1 [1.2] vs 2 [1.4] days, respectively, $P = .07$), duration of thoracic epidural analgesia (2 [2.3] vs 3 [2.5] days, respectively, $P = .07$), or hospital stay (4 [4.5] vs 4.5 [4.7] days, respectively, $P = .12$).

In a single-institution study of 113 patients undergoing lobectomy, segmentectomy, or wedge resection by 2 surgeons, Fabian and colleagues[16] randomized 50 consecutive patients to receive fibrin sealant (fibrinogen, procoagulants, aprotinin, thrombin, and calcium) sprayed to raw and stapled lung surfaces (treatment) and 50 patients not (control) (evidence grade 2A). A blinded observer made all postoperative assessments. Comparing treatment with control groups, fibrin sealant had a decreased mean duration of air leak (1.1 [range, 0–10] vs 3.1 [0–19] days, respectively, variability not stated, $P = .005$) mean time to chest tube removal (5 vs 3.5 days, respectively, measure of variability not given, $P = .02$), and overall occurrence of air leak (68% vs 34%, respectively, measure of variability not given, $P = .001$). However, hospital stay (4.6 vs 4.9 days, respectively, measure of variability not given, $P = .3$), and percentage of patients discharged with a chest tube (2% vs 16%, respectively, measure of variability not given, $P = .3$) were similar.

*Metastasectomy—precision cautery* There has been 1 randomized study evaluating fibrin sealant in pulmonary metastasectomy (see **Table 2**). In a single-institution study of 100 consecutive patients undergoing cautery excision of pulmonary metastases, Brega Massone and colleagues[17] randomized equal numbers to receive fibrin sealant (fibrinogen, factor XIII, fibronectin, plasminogen, aprotinin, thrombin, and calcium) sprayed onto metastasectomy site (treatment) and cautery alone (control) (evidence grade 2C). Paradoxically, plasminogen was used in this commercial preparation. Comparing treatment with control groups, fibrin sealant had a decreased duration of air leak (2.6 ± 1.7 vs 7.8 ± 8.5 days, respectively, $P<.001$), mean time to chest tube removal (4.5 ± 1.8 vs 9.5 ± 8.3 days, respectively, $P<.001$), and hospital stay (6.5 ± 1.8 days vs 11.5 ± 8.3 days, respectively, $P<.001$), but distribution of these data in the control group is skewed, so test statistics are suspect.

*Complications*
As with all human blood products, transmission of infections is a consideration. In lung surgery, this complication has not been attributed to fibrin sealants. Bovine-derived thrombin and aprotinin could potentially transmit bovine spongiform encephalitis and may, after repeated exposure, produce anaphylactic reactions. There has been a single report of anaphylaxis with use of fibrin sealant in pulmonary surgery.[18] After 7 applications of fibrin sealant following myringoplasty, its use during lobectomy was associated with severe hypotension and 2 days of hemodynamic instability. Immunoglobulin E (IgE) antibodies targeted bovine aprotinin as the source of this allergic reaction.

*Recommendations*
Fibrin sealants variably reduce the magnitude, occurrence, and duration of air leak following pulmonary surgery (see **Table 2**). These inconsistent improvements did not reliably translate into reduced duration of chest tube drainage or hospital stay (see **Table 2**). Use of fibrin sealants has not been associated with increased or specific complications. Cost studies have not been performed. Routine use of fibrin sealant in pulmonary surgery, prophylactically or for air leaks present at operation, is not supported by this evidence-based literature review.

## Synthetic Sealant

### Glutaraldehyde-albumin sealant
Glutaraldehyde is a preservative and disinfectant that exerts its action by cross-linking proteins. It has been infrequently used as a pulmonary sealant, experimentally and clinically.

### Experimental evidence
In sheep, application of glutaraldehyde-albumin sealant to suture closure of lung incisions produced a granulomatous reaction 4 weeks postoperatively; this was not seen with suture closure.[19] No air leaks occurred in either group. However, at 12 weeks there were few remnants of sealant surrounded by fibrous scar tissue, with no evidence of granuloma. In rats, a glutaraldehyde-based sealant was superior to fibrin sealant or cyanoacrylate-based sealant in control of air leak from thermally injured lungs.[20] Glutaraldehyde sealant tightly adhered to the damaged lung surface, unlike the other sealants, and complete pneumostasis was achieved. At 20 days after surgery, it was encased and fragmented and, by 40 days, partially absorbed. In pigs, the composition and preparation of experimental glutaraldehyde-albumin sealants was found to influence cohesive and adhesive strengths and thus quality of air leak control.[21] The glutaraldehyde-based sealant with the highest cohesive and adhesive strengths was the most effective lung sealant.

### Clinical evidence
**Pulmonary resection** There has been 1 randomized study evaluating glutaraldehyde-albumin sealant in pulmonary resection (**Table 3**). In a single-institution study of 52 patients undergoing pulmonary resection by 1 of 3 surgeons and judged intraoperatively to have an air leak, Tansley and colleagues[22] randomized 25 patients to receive a mixture of glutaraldehyde and bovine serum albumin applied to air leaks from the pulmonary surface (treatment) and 27 not (control) (evidence grade 1B) (see **Table 3**). Comparing treatment with control groups, the sealant group was reported to have shorter duration of air leak

**Table 3**
**Synthetic sealants: findings in RCTs**

| Sealant/ First Author | Reduction in Air Leak | | | Reduction in: | | Difference in: | | Evidence Grade |
| --- | --- | --- | --- | --- | --- | --- | --- | --- |
| | Magnitude | Incidence | Duration | Chest Tube Duration | Hospital Stay | Cost | Complications | |
| Glutaraldehyde | | | | | | | | |
| Tansley et al[22] | NS | ↓ | ↓ | ↓ | ↓ | NS | ± | 1B |
| Polyethylene glycol | | | | | | | | |
| Macchiarini et al[23] | NS | ↓ | ± | ± | ± | ± | ± | 2A |
| Porte et al[24] | ↓ | ↓ 4 day ± 6 day | ↓ | NR | ± | NS | ± | 2B |
| Wain et al[25] | NS | ↓ | ↓ | ± | ± | NS | ± | 1B |
| Allen et al[26] | NS | ↓ | ± | ± | ↓ | NS | ± | 1B |
| D'Andrilli et al[27] | NS | ↓ | ↓ | NR | ± | NS | ± | 2B |

*Abbreviations:* ↓, decrease; ±, no difference; NR, not reported; NS, not studied.

(median [interquartile range] 1 [0–2] vs 4 [2–6] days, respectively, $P<.001$), shorter duration of chest tube drainage (4 [3–4] vs 5 [4–6] days, respectively, $P = .01$), and shorter hospitalization (6 [5–7] vs 7 [7–10] days, respectively, $P = .004$).

### Complications

Although other aldehydes, such as formaldehyde, have been associated with increased upper respiratory tract cancers and leukemia, glutaraldehyde in a small series has not been found to have such associations.[28] Release of glutaraldehyde from albumin-glutaraldehyde tissue adhesive has been shown to cause in vitro and in vivo cellular toxicity.[29] Pulmonary fibrosis has been reported as a complication of glutaraldehyde sealant.[30] In a pulmonary sealant trial using bovine serum albumin, increased antibovine serum albumin antibodies were reported in patients receiving sealant during pulmonary resection, but this was not associated with any detectable clinical events.[31]

### Polyethylene glycol sealants

Unlike other sealants, polyethylene glycol–based sealants do not form a covalent bond with tissue, but create a mechanical bond by interpolation of the sealant into irregular surfaces. These hydrogels absorb water for 24 hours and therefore can tolerate moist surfaces, but not bleeding. The sealant is degraded by hydrolysis.

### Experimental evidence

In pigs, no air leak was detected from bronchial stumps closed with staples and coated with sealant or with sealant alone.[23] In rats, a polyethylene glycol sealant was superior to fibrin sealant in sealing pleural defects.[32] Higher burst pressures were measured for the polyethylene glycol sealant at time 0 and day 3, but not day 7. In dogs, a combination of fibrin and polyethylene glycol sealant was superior to fibrin sealant alone or fibrin-glue–coated collagen fleece in sealing pleural defects.[33] In this combination sealant, resistance to air leak with increasing inflation pressure was better at 5 minutes, 1 hour, and 3 hours after application, and increased with time.

### Clinical evidence

*Pulmonary resection* There have been 5 randomized studies evaluating polyethylene glycol–based sealants in pulmonary resections (see **Table 3**). In a 2-institution study of 26 patients with an air leak undergoing lobectomy or less, Macchiarini and colleagues[23] randomized 15 patients to receive a light-activated polyethylene glycol–based sealant applied to all surgical sites, excluding the bronchial stump (treatment) and 11 not (control) (evidence grade 2A). Comparing treatment with control groups, the sealant group was reported to have improved sealing of intraoperative air leak (100% vs 18%, respectively, $P = .001$) and postoperative freedom from air leak (77% vs 9%, respectively, $P = .001$). However, duration of chest tube drainage, hospitalization, and cost were similar.

In a single-institution study of 124 patients with an air leak undergoing lobectomy by 1 of 2 surgeons, Porte and colleagues[24] randomized 59 patients with moderate to severe intraoperative air leak to receive a light-activated polyethylene glycol polymer sealant applied to all leaking or at-risk surgical sites (treatment) and 61 patients not (control). Comparing treatment with control groups, the sealant group was reported to have reduced mean air leak volume after treatment (38 ± 43 vs 60 ± 53 mL, respectively, $P$ = .04, but distribution of data is skewed and statistical tests inappropriate), reduced mean time to last air leak (34 vs 63 hours, respectively, $P$ = .01), and increased percentage of patients free of air leak at day 4 (87% vs 59%, respectively, $P$ = .002). However, percentage of patients free of air leak at day 6 (87% vs 78%, respectively, $P$ = NS) and in-hospital stay (9.2 ± 5.0 vs 8.6 ± 3.3 days, respectively, $P$ = NS) were similar. Empyema not seen in controls was reported in 4 treatment patients. In an additional 20 treatment patients, computed tomography findings were suggestive of empyema, which cleared in 10.

In a multi-institutional study of 172 consecutive patients undergoing bilobectomy or less, Wain and colleagues[25] randomized 125 to receive a light-activated polyethylene glycol polymer sealant applied to leaking sites (treatment) and 55 patients not (control) (evidence grade 1B). Comparing treatment with control groups, the sealant group was reported to have increased percentage of patients without air leak at skin closure (92% vs 29%, respectively, $P \leq$ .001), increased freedom from air leak during hospitalization (39% vs 11%, respectively, $P \leq$ .001), and reduced time from skin closure to last observable air leak (31 ± 5.0 vs 52 ± 12 hours, respectively, $P$ = .006). However, duration of chest tube drainage and hospital stay were similar.

In a 5-institution study of 161 patients with an air leak undergoing bilobectomy or less, Allen and colleagues[26] randomized 95 to receive polyethylene glycol polymer sealant applied to leaking sites (treatment) and 53 patients not (control) (evidence grade 1B). The primary end point, percentage of patients free of air leak at 1 month follow-up, was realized in 35% of treatment patients and 14% of controls ($P$ = .005). Comparing treatment with control groups, the sealant group was reported to have shorter median hospital stay (6 [range, 3–23] vs 7 [range, 4–38] days, respectively, $P$ = .03). Secondary end points (mortality, morbidity, duration of chest tube drainage, and immune response) were similar.

In a single-institution study of 203 patients with an air leak undergoing bilobectomy or less, D'Andrilli and colleagues[27] randomized 102 to receive polyethylene glycol sealant applied to leaking sites (treatment) and 101 patients not (control) (evidence grade 2B). Comparing treatment with control groups, the sealant group was reported

to have decreased intraoperative air leak occurrence (85% vs 59%, respectively, $P$<.001), 24- and 48-hour postoperative air leak occurrence (20% vs 41%, $P$ = .001; and 24% vs 42%, respectively, $P$ = .006), and duration of air leak (3.5 ± 1.7 vs 4.2 ± 2.4 days, respectively, $P$ = .01 [95% confidence interval (CI) 0.13, 1.27 for difference]). Duration of hospital stay was similar.

## Complications
There have been no reports of specific complications associated with polyethylene glycol–based sealants in pulmonary surgery.

## Recommendations
Compared with fibrin sealants, synthetic sealants more reliably decrease magnitude, occurrence, and duration of air leak. However, this does not result in reduced duration of chest tube drainage or hospital stay. Cost savings were not seen in the only study evaluating cost. Evidence-based literature does not support routine use of synthetic sealants, prophylactically or for established air leaks, in pulmonary surgery (see **Table 3**). However, this recommendation may be moot because polyethylene glycol–based sealants are no longer produced or available in the United States.

## Collagen fleece–bound fibrin sealants
Fibrin-coated collagen sheets were introduced as hemostatic agents in vascular, liver, and kidney surgery. This refinement of fibrin sealants has been proposed as a sealant for air leaks. Considered a dual agent, a potential advantage is control of air leaks from a bleeding surface.

## Experimental evidence
In pigs, collagen fleece–bound fibrin sealant was no more effective than electrocautery in reducing magnitude of air leak from a standardized pulmonary injury.[34] Adhesion score was similar 8 weeks after surgery. Method of application may determine the ability of fibrin sealant to control air leak. In dogs, the sealing effect of collagen fleece–bound fibrin sealants was inferior to fibrin sealant.[8]

## Clinical evidence
**Pulmonary resections** There have been 5 randomized studies evaluating collagen fleece–bound fibrin sealants in pulmonary resections (**Table 4**). In a 5-institution study of 189 consecutive patients undergoing lobectomy, Lang and colleagues[35] randomized 96 patients to receive equine collagen fleece coated with human fibrinogen and collagen to all surgical sites (treatment) and 93 not (control) (evidence grade 2A). Comparing treatment with

**Table 4**
**Fleece-bound sealants: findings in RCTs**

| First Author | Reduction in Air Leak | | | Reduction in: | | Difference in: | | |
| | Magnitude | Incidence | Duration | Chest Tube Duration | Hospital Stay | Cost | Complications | Evidence Grade |
|---|---|---|---|---|---|---|---|---|
| Lang et al[35] | ↓ Intraoperatively ± ± Postoperatively | ± | ± | NS | NS | NS | ± | 2A |
| Anegg et al[36,37] | ↓ | ± | ± | ↓ | ↓ | ± | ± | 2C |
| Droghetti et al[38] | ↓ | ↓ | ↓ | ± | ± | ± | ± | 2A |
| Rena et al[39] | ↓ | ↓ | ↓ | ↓ | ↓ | NS | ± | 2B |
| Marta et al[40] | ? | ↓ | ↓ | ? | ? | ? | ± | ? |

*Abbreviations:* ↓, decrease; ±, no difference; ?, not yet published; NS, not studied.

control groups, the sealant group was reported to have decreased magnitude of air leak intraoperatively by 1 or 2 levels on a 4-level air leak scale (74% vs 51%, respectively, $P = .015$). However, mean magnitude of intensity of air leak postoperatively measured by a 9-level air leak meter ($0.8 \pm 1.7$ vs $1.3 \pm 2.8$, respectively, $P = .07$), occurrence of air leak at 48 hours (34% vs 37%, respectively, $P = .8$), and duration of air leak ($1.7 \pm 1.2$ vs $2.0 \pm 1.8$, respectively, $P = .07$) were similar.

In a single-institution study of 152 consecutive patients with an air leak undergoing lobectomy or segmentectomy, Anegg and colleagues[36] randomized 75 patients to receive equine collagen fleece coated with human fibrinogen and collagen to all pulmonary surfaces with air leak (treatment) and 77 not (control) (evidence grade 2C). All comparisons were done with $t$-tests, despite some time-related measures and skewed data, that, combined with inconsistently reported variability, make the analysis difficult to interpret. Comparing treatment with control groups, the sealant group was reported to have decreased mean magnitude of air leak intraoperatively (153 [range, 10–450] vs 251 [range, 15–970] mL/min, respectively) and at day 1 postoperatively (44 vs 86 mL/min, respectively, variability not stated, $P = .02$), but not at day 2 postoperatively (20 vs 42 mL/min, respectively, variability not stated, $P = .2$). Duration of air leak was similar. Comparing treatment with control groups, the sealant group was reported to have decreased duration of chest tube drainage (5.1 vs 6.3 days, respectively, variability not stated, $P = .02$) and hospital stay (6.2 vs 7.7 days, respectively, variability not stated, $P = .01$). In a secondary analysis of this study, the increased cost of the collagen fleece–bound fibrin sealant, a tenfold increase in technical costs, was offset by the 1.5-day reduction in hospital

stay.[37] Use of sealant was reported to reduce costs by €99.

In a single-institution study of 40 consecutive patients undergoing lobectomy, Droghetti and colleagues[38] randomized 20 to receive equine collagen fleece coated with human fibrinogen and collagen to all fissures divided by electrocautery (treatment) and 20 with stapler division of fissures (control) (evidence grade 2B). Comparing treatment with control groups, the sealant group had a decreased magnitude of air leak ($P = .03$), occurrence of air leak at 48 hours (50% vs 95%, respectively, $P = .001$), and mean duration of air leak (1.7 [range, 0–10] vs 4.5 [range, 0–16] days, respectively, $P = .003$). Durations of chest tube drainage and hospital stay were similar. Mean technical costs were higher in the sealant group (€630 vs €435, respectively, no variability stated, $P = .001$), but overall hospital costs were similar.

In a single-institution study of 60 consecutive patients with chronic obstructive pulmonary disease and lung cancer undergoing lobectomy, Rena and colleagues[39] intraoperatively randomized 30 patients to receive equine collagen fleece coated with human fibrinogen and collagen to all fissures divided by electrocautery (treatment) and 30 with stapler division of fissures (control) (evidence grade 2B). Interpretation of results is difficult because skewed data were interpreted by parametric analyses. Comparing treatment with control groups, the sealant group had a decreased magnitude of air leak ($182 \pm 162$ vs $293 \pm 209$ mL/min, respectively, $P = .03$), occurrence of air leak immediately postoperatively and at 1 day and 3 days postoperatively (immediate 70% vs 90%, respectively, $P = NS$; 1 day 63% vs 90%, respectively, $P = .03$; and 3 days 20% vs 50%, respectively, $P = .03$), mean duration of air leak ($1.6 \pm 2.0$ vs $4.3 \pm 4.1$ days, respectively,

$P = .001$), mean chest tube duration (3.5 ± 1.6 vs 5.9 ± 3.7 days, respectively, $P = .002$), and hospital stay (5.9 ± 1.1 days vs 7.5 ± 3.2 days, respectively, $P = .01$).

In a 12-institution study of 301 patients undergoing lobectomy with grade 1 or 2 air leaks, Marta and colleagues[40] intraoperatively randomized 149 patients to receive equine collagen fleece coated with human fibrinogen and collagen to all fissures divided by stapler (treatment) and 150 with stapler division of fissures (control) (evidence grade ?). Only a published abstract is available at the time of writing this manuscript. Comparing treatment with control groups, the sealant group had a decreased occurrence of air leak immediately postoperatively (32% vs 58%, respectively, $P = .02$), duration of air leak ($P = .03$), and percentage of patients free of air leak at discharge (30% vs 19%, respectively, $P = .02$). No other results were available at the time of writing this manuscript.

## Complications

Equine-derived collagen on re-exposure could theoretically produce anaphylactic reactions. As with all human blood products, transmission of infections is a consideration. In lung surgery, these complications have not been attributed to collagen fleece–bound fibrin sealants.

## Recommendations

Despite being the most recent experience, studies of collagen fleece–bound fibrin sealants are, to date, the least well conducted and analyzed. Evidence-based literature does not support the routine use of these sealants in pulmonary surgery (see **Table 4**).

## STAPLE-LINE BUTTRESSING

In the early to mid-1990s, resurgence and aggressive application of surgery for emphysema produced an epidemic of air leaks complicating LVRS. In this setting, many air leaks result from resection of fragile, damaged, emphysematous pulmonary parenchyma. The complication is magnified by long resection lines necessary to remove large portions of the most diseased lung. To deal with this almost universal complication, Cooper[41] reintroduced and refined the concept of staple-line buttressing (evidence grade 2C). Borrowed from vascular surgery and described before the introduction of LVRS (evidence grade 2C),[42–46] buttressing theoretically supports the emphysematous tissues and provides an anchor into which staples can be fired. By sandwiching lung between buttress materials, the forces produced on inspiration are distributed along the length and depth of the staple line. These buttressing techniques were rapidly adopted with incomplete supporting evidence. Only late in the LVRS experience did some data become available.

### Experimental evidence

Murray and colleagues[47] measured the airway pressure necessary to produce staple-line air leaks in cadaver lungs. Two types of linear cutting staplers were used to produce nonbuttressed and buttressed staple lines. Buttress material was bovine pericardium (BP) or expanded polytetra-fluoroethylene (ePTFE). At airway pressure of 15 cm $H_2O$, no air leaks were seen. Air leaks from nonbuttressed staple lines increased exponentially after this pressure, with 100% staple-line leakage at airway pressure greater than 60 cm $H_2O$ (**Fig. 1**). The percentage of buttressed staple lines developing air leaks increased linearly until more than 55 cm $H_2O$ (burst pressure); thereafter, 100% developed air leaks (see **Fig. 1**). Airway pressure (95% CI) when half of staple lines leaked was 20 to 25 cm $H_2O$ for nonbuttressed staple lines, 40 to 55 cm $H_2O$ for BP-buttressed staple lines, and at least 55 cm $H_2O$ for ePTFE-buttressed staple lines. For this study, 2 different staplers were used; there was no difference in air leaks between them.

In dogs, nonbuttressed staple lines were inferior to 3 types of buttressed staple lines.[48] Mean pressure at which air leak occurred was 10.8 cm $H_2O$ higher with buttressing. There was no difference among BP, ePTFE, or prototype ePTFE buttresses.

In pigs, 4 types of buttressing materials were compared and no buttressing served as control.[49]

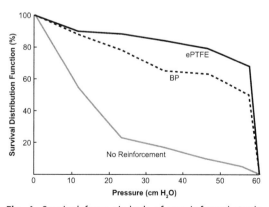

**Fig. 1.** Survival from air leak of unreinforced staple lines and staples reinforced with ePTFE or BP. Survival or freedom from air leaks was significantly different for all comparisons. (*Adapted from* Murray KD, Ho CH, Hsia JY, et al. The influence of pulmonary staple line reinforcement on air leaks. Chest 2002;122:2148; with permission.)

Along with BP and ePTFE, a bioabsorbable material, polyglycolic acid-trimethylene carbonate, and porcine small intestinal submucosa (SIS) were studied. No air leaks were seen in any staple line (including control) at airway pressures less than 20 cm $H_2O$. Unlike other experimental studies, no buttressing material except SIS ($P<.04$) was better than none at preventing air leaks (**Fig. 2**).

In the lung, tissue response to BP and ePTFE are different. In dogs, BP incited focal chronic inflammation at 30 days; however, no tissue incorporation was seen up to 167 days after surgery.[50] In contrast, ePTFE incited minimal inflammation and had increasing tissue incorporation over time ($P>.0001$). Despite this difference, there were no air leaks, staple-line disruptions, or infections in either study group.

### Clinical evidence

**LVRS** Three randomized studies have been conducted in patients undergoing LVRS. In a 2-institution study of 123 consecutive patients, Hazelrigg and colleagues[51] randomized 58 patients to receive BP-buttressed staple lines and 65 not (control) (evidence grade 2C). Patients with buttressed staple lines had a shorter duration of chest tube drainage compared with controls (7.9 vs 10.4 days, respectively, $P = .04$) and shorter hospital stay (8.6 vs 11.4 days, respectively, $P = .03$). Hospital costs were similar between groups; however, data were skewed, so true results are not interpretable.

In a single-institution study of 60 consecutive patients, Santambrogio and colleagues[52] randomized an equal number of patients to receive BP-buttressed staple lines and not (control) (evidence grade 2B). Air leak duration did not differ between groups. However, air leak duration increased with increasing radiographic emphysema score ($P<.001$). In subgroup analysis, air leak duration was significantly reduced only in patients with the most severe emphysema score who received buttressed staple lines ($P = .02$).

In a 3-institution study of 74 consecutive patients, Stammberger and colleagues[53] randomized 32 patients to receive BP-buttressed staple lines and 33 not (control) (evidence grade 2A). Median duration of air leak was shorter in the buttressed group compared with controls (0 [range, 0–28] vs 4 [range, 0–27] days, respectively, $P<.001$), as was median duration of chest tube drainage (5 [range, 1–35] vs 7.5 [range, 2–29] days, respectively, $P = .04$). This difference did not result in shorter hospital stay ($P = .14$).

In an observational study of 57 consecutive patients, Fischel and McKenna[54] compared BP-buttressed staple lines in 1 lung with bovine collagen (BC)–buttressed staples in the contralateral lung (evidence grade 2B). There was no difference in time to chest tube removal with either technique. However, use of BC was associated with an 80% lower cost. In another observational study of 10 patients undergoing LVRS, BP-buttressed stapling in 1 lung was compared with bovine serum albumin- and glutaraldehyde-coated staple lines in the contralateral lung (evidence grade 2C).[55] In this underpowered study, no difference was found in duration of air leak or amount or duration of chest tube drainage.

A secondary analysis of National Emphysema Treatment Trial (NETT) data focused on air leaks (evidence grade 1B).[56] Data were available in 552 of 580 patients treated with bilateral stapled LVRS. Ninety percent experienced air leaks within 30 days of surgery. Only patient factors, lower diffusing capacity, upper-lobe emphysema, and important pleural adhesions were predictors of air leaks. Surgical factors such as staple-line buttressing, stapler brand, or intraoperative adjunctive procedures were not associated with fewer or less-prolonged air leaks ($P\geq.2$).

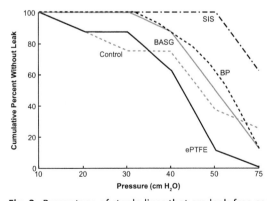

**Fig. 2.** Percentage of staple lines that are leak free as a function of pressure (cm $H_2O$). Leak occurrence was substantially improved with reinforcement of the staple lines with SIS. BASG, bioabsorbable Seamguard. (*Adapted from* Downey D, Harre JG, Pratt JW. Functional comparison of staple line reinforcements in lung resection. Ann Thorac Surg 2006;82:1881; with permission.)

### Pulmonary Resection

Two randomized studies have examined the effect of staple-line buttressing in patients undergoing pulmonary resections. In a single-institution study, Venuta and colleagues[57] randomized 30 consecutive patients with incomplete pulmonary fissures undergoing lobectomy into 3 equal-size groups (evidence grade 2B). Three techniques were used for fissure control: BP-buttressed staple lines;

nonbuttressed staple lines; and old-fashioned cautery, clamps, and silk ties (control). In patients with buttressed staple closure of incomplete fissures, duration of air leaks ($2 \pm 0.94$, $5.3 \pm 2.0$, $5.3 \pm 1.7$ days, respectively) and hospital stay ($4.4 \pm 0.96$, $7.8 \pm 2.1$, $7.2 \pm 1.5$ days, respectively) were shorter ($P > .0001$).

In a 2-institution study of 80 consecutive patients undergoing lobectomy or segmentectomy, Miller and colleagues[58] randomized 40 patients to staple-line buttressing with BP and 40 not (control) group (evidence grade 2B). Duration of air leak, duration of chest tube drainage, length of intensive care unit (ICU) stay, length of hospital stay, and cost were similar between groups, but portions of the data were skewed, so information is difficult to interpret.

## Complications

BP buttressing has been associated with unique complications. It has produced symptomatic mass lesions suggestive of malignancy or inhaled foreign body.[59] Hemoptysis and expectoration of staples (metalloptysis) and pieces of BP have been reported.[60–64] Better tissue incorporation of ePTFE may account for the infrequent complications reported with the use of this buttressing material.[65]

## Recommendations

Staple-line buttressing in experimental and clinical applications has produced variable and equivocal effects on air leak reduction. In LVRS, patient factors, not surgical techniques, seem to be the strongest determinants of air leak. Routine use of staple-line buttressing in pulmonary surgery is not supported by evidence-based literature. If used, it should be on a per-patient basis with the realization that its effectiveness is hypothetical. BP is associated with specific unique complications that make it the least desirable buttressing material.

## SUMMARY

An evidence-based analysis of the current literature does not support routine use, prophylactically or for air leaks present at operation, of sealants (median evidence grade 2B) or buttressing material (median evidence grade 2B) in pulmonary surgery.

## REFERENCES

1. Rice TW, Kirby TJ. Prolonged air leak. Chest Surg Clin N Am 1992;2:803–11.

2. Rice TW, Okereke IC, Blackstone EH. Persistent air-leak following pulmonary resection. Chest Surg Clin N Am 2002;12:529–39.

3. Guyatt G, Gutterman D, Baumann MH, et al. Grading strength of recommendations and quality of evidence in clinical guidelines: report from an American College of Chest Physicians Task Force. Chest 2006;129:174–81.

4. Türk R, Weidringer JW, Hartel W, et al. Closure of lung leaks by fibrin gluing. Experimental investigations and clinical experience. J Thorac Cardiovasc Surg 1983;31:185–6.

5. Bergsland J, Kalmbach T, Balu D, et al. Fibrin seal—an alternative to suture repair in experimental pulmonary surgery. J Surg Res 1986;40:340–5.

6. McCarthy PM, Trastek VF, Bell DG, et al. The effectiveness of fibrin glue sealant for reducing experimental pulmonary air leak. Ann Thorac Surg 1988;45:203–5.

7. Kjaergard HK, Pedersen JH, Krasnik M, et al. Prevention of air leakage by spraying Vivostat fibrin sealant after lung resection in pigs. Chest 2000;117:1124–7.

8. Kawamura M, Gika M, Izumi Y, et al. The sealing effect of fibrin glue against alveolar air leakage evaluated up to 48 h; comparison between different methods of application. Eur J Cardiothorac Surg 2005;28:39–42.

9. Moser C, Opitz I, Zhai W, et al. Autologous fibrin sealant reduces the incidence of prolonged air leak and duration of chest tube drainage after lung volume reduction surgery: a prospective randomized blinded study. J Thorac Cardiovasc Surg 2008;136:843–9.

10. Fleisher AG, Evans KG, Nelems B, et al. Effect of routine fibrin glue use on the duration of air leaks after lobectomy. Ann Thorac Surg 1990;49:133–4.

11. Wurtz A, Chambon JP, Sobecki L, et al. Utilisation d'une colle biologique en chirurgie d'exérèse pulmonaire partielle. Ann Chir 1990;45:719–23.

12. Wurtz A, Bambiez JP, Saudemont A. Evaluation de l'efficacité d'une colle fibrine en chirurgie d'exérèse pulmonaire partielle. Résultats d'un nouvel essai contrôlé chez 50 malades. Lyon Chir 1992;88:368–71 [in French].

13. Mouritzen C, Dromer M, Keinecke HO. The effect of fibrin glueing to seal bronchial and alveolar leakages after pulmonary resections and decortications. Eur J Cardiothorac Surg 1993;7:75–80.

14. Wong K, Goldstraw P. Effect of fibrin glue in the reduction of postthoracotomy alveolar air leak. Ann Thorac Surg 1997;64:979–81.

15. Belboul A, Dernevik L, Aljassim O, et al. The effect of autologous fibrin sealant (Vivostat) on morbidity after pulmonary lobectomy: a prospective randomised, blinded study. Eur J Cardiothorac Surg 2004;26:1187–91.

16. Fabian T, Federico JA, Ponn RB. Fibrin glue in pulmonary resection: a prospective, randomized, blinded study. Ann Thorac Surg 2003;75:1587–92.

17. Brega Massone PP, Magnani B, Conti B, et al. Cauterization versus fibrin glue for aerostasis in precision resections for secondary lung tumors. Ann Surg Oncol 2003;10:441–6.

18. Shirai T, Shimota H, Chida K, et al. Anaphylaxis to aprotinin in fibrin sealant. Intern Med 2005;44:1088–9.

19. Herget GW, Kassa M, Riede UN, et al. Experimental use of an albumin-glutaraldehyde tissue adhesive for sealing pulmonary parenchyma and bronchial anastomoses. Eur J Cardiothorac Surg 2001;19:4–9.

20. Kodama K, Doi O, Higashiyama M, et al. Pneumostatic effect of gelatin-resorcinol formaldehyde-glutaraldehyde glue on thermal injury of the lung: an experimental study on rats. Eur J Cardiothorac Surg 1997;11:333–7.

21. Browdie DA, Cox D. Tests of experimental tissue adhesive sealants: analysis of strength effects in relation to tissue adhesive sealant standards. Tex Heart Inst J 2007;34:313–7.

22. Tansley P, Al-Mulhim F, Lim E, et al. A prospective, randomized, controlled trial of the effectiveness of BioGlue in treating alveolar air leaks. J Thorac Cardiovasc Surg 2006;132:105–12.

23. Macchiarini P, Wain J, Almy S, et al. Experimental and clinical evaluation of a new synthetic, absorbable sealant to reduce air leaks in thoracic operations. J Thorac Cardiovasc Surg 1999;117:751–8.

24. Porte HL, Jany T, Akkad R, et al. Randomized controlled trial of a synthetic sealant for preventing alveolar air leaks after lobectomy. Ann Thorac Surg 2001;71:1618–22.

25. Wain JC, Kaiser LR, Johnstone DW, et al. Trial of a novel synthetic sealant in preventing air leaks after lung resection. Ann Thorac Surg 2001;71:1623–9.

26. Allen MS, Wood DE, Hawkinson RW, et al. Prospective randomized study evaluating a biodegradeable polymeric sealant for sealing intraoperative air leaks that occur during pulmonary resection. Ann Thorac Surg 2004;77:1792–801.

27. D'Andrilli AD, Andreetti C, Ibrahim M, et al. A prospective randomized study to assess the efficacy of a surgical sealant to treat air leaks in lung surgery. Eur J Cardiothorac Surg 2009;35:817–21.

28. Collins JJ, Burns C, Spencer P, et al. Respiratory cancer risks among workers with glutaraldehyde exposure. J Occup Environ Med 2006;48:199–203.

29. Fürst W, Banerjee A. Release of glutaraldehyde from an albumin-glutaraldehyde tissue adhesive causes significant in vitro and in vivo toxicity. Ann Thorac Surg 2005;79:1522–8.

30. Haj-Yahia S, Mittal T, Birks E, et al. Lung fibrosis as a potential complication of the hemostatic tissue sealant, biologic glue (Bioglue). J Thorac Cardiovasc Surg 2007;133:1387–8.

31. Mogues T, Li J, Coburn J, et al. IgG antibodies against bovine serum albumin in humans—their prevalence and response to exposure to bovine serum albumin. J Immunol Methods 2005;300:1–11.

32. Kobayachi H, Sokino T, Nakamura T, et al. In vivo evaluation of a new sealant material on a rat lung air leak model. J Biomed Mater Res 2001;58:658–65.

33. Gika M, Kawamura M, Izumi Y, et al. The short-term efficacy of fibrin glue combined with absorptive sheet material in visceral pleural defect repair. Interact Cardiovasc Thorac Surg 2007;6:12–5.

34. Izbicki JR, Kreusser T, Meier M, et al. Fibrin-glue-coated collagen fleece in lung surgery–experimental comparison with infrared coagulation and clinical experience. Thorac Cardiovasc Surg 1994;42:306–9.

35. Lang G, Csekeo A, Stamatis G, et al. Efficacy and safety of topical application of human fibrinogen/thrombin-coated collagen patch (TachoComb) for treatment of air leakage after standard lobectomy. Eur J Cardiothorac Surg 2004;25:160–6.

36. Anegg U, Lindenmann J, Matzi V, et al. Efficiency of fleece-bound sealing (TachoSil) of air leaks in lung surgery: a prospective randomised trial. Eur J Cardiothorac Surg 2007;31:198–202.

37. Anegg U, Rychlik R, Smolle-Jüttner F. Do the benefits of shorter hospital stay associated with the use of fleece-bound sealing outweigh the costs of the materials? Interact Cardiovasc Thorac Surg 2008;7:292–6.

38. Droghetti A, Schiavini A, Muriana P, et al. A prospective randomized trial comparing completion technique of fissures for lobectomy: stapler versus precision dissection and sealant. J Thorac Cardiovasc Surg 2008;136:383–91.

39. Rena O, Papalia E, Mineo TC, et al. Air-leak management after upper lobectomy in patients with fused fissure and chronic obstructive pulmonary disease: a pilot trial comparing sealant and standard treatment. Interact Cardiovasc Thorac Surg 2009;9:973–7.

40. Marta GM, Facciolo F, Ladegaard L, et al. Sustained air sealing efficacy of Tachosil in pulmonary lobectomy. In: Programs and abstracts of the 46th Annual Meeting of the Society of Thoracic Surgeons. Elsevier Science, Inc, Lauderdale (FL), 2010.

41. Cooper JD. Technique to reduce air leaks after resection of emphysematous lung. Ann Thorac Surg 1994;57:1038–9.

42. Parmar JM, Hubbard WG, Matthews HR. Teflon strip pneumostasis for excision of giant emphysematous bullae. Thorax 1987;42:144–8.

43. Cole PH. Stapling air leaks. Chest 1988;94:1118.

44. Juettner FM, Kohek P, Pinter H, et al. Reinforced staple line in severely emphysematous lungs. J Thorac Cardiovasc Surg 1989;97:362–3.

45. Fulton RL, Dickson M. A useful technique for closure of pulmonary lacerations. Ann Thorac Surg 1990;50:149–50.

46. Vincent JG. Reinforcement of pulmonary paren-chymal suture [comment]. Ann Thorac Surg 1991; 51:523–4.

47. Murray KD, Ho CH, Hsia JY, et al. The influence of pulmonary staple line reinforcement on air leaks. Chest 2002;122:2146–9.

48. Roberson LD, Netherland DE, Dhillon R, et al. Air leaks after surgical stapling in lung resection: a comparison between stapling alone and stapling with staple-line reinforcement materials in a canine model. J Thorac Cardiovasc Surg 1998;116:353–4.

49. Downey DM, Harre JG, Pratt JW. Functional compar-ison of staple line reinforcements in lung resection. Ann Thorac Surg 2006;82:1880–3.

50. Vaughn CC, Vaughn PL, Vaughn CC 3rd, et al. Tissue response to biomaterials used for staple-line reinforcement in lung resection: a comparison between expanded polytetrafluoroethylene and bovine pericardium. Eur J Cardiothorac Surg 1998; 13:259–65.

51. Hazelrigg SR, Boley TM, Naunheim KS, et al. Effect of bovine pericardial strips on air leak after stapled pulmonary resection. Ann Thorac Surg 1997;63: 1573–5.

52. Santambrogio L, Nosotti M, Baisi A, et al. Buttress-ing staple lines with bovine pericardium in lung resection for bullous emphysema. Scand Cardio-vasc J 1998;32:297–9.

53. Stammberger U, Klepetko W, Stamatis G, et al. But-tressing the staple line in lung volume reduction surgery: a randomized three-center study. Ann Thor-ac Surg 2000;70:1820–5.

54. Fischel RJ, McKenna RJ Jr. Bovine pericardium versus bovine collagen to buttress staples for lung reduction operations. Ann Thorac Surg 1998;65: 217–9.

55. Rathinam S, Naidu BV, Nanjaiah P, et al. BioGlue and Peri-strips in lung volume reduction surgery: pilot

56. DeCamp MM, Blackstone EH, Naunheim KS, et al. NETT Research Group. Patient and surgical factors influencing air leak after lung volume reduction surgery: lessons learned from the National Emphysema Treat-ment Trial. Ann Thorac Surg 2006;82:197–206.

57. Venuta F, Rendina EA, De Giacomo T, et al. Tech-nique to reduce air leaks after pulmonary lobectomy. Eur J Cardiothorac Surg 1998;13:361–4.

58. Miller JI Jr, Landreneau RJ, Wright CE, et al. A comparative study of buttressed versus nonbut-tressed staple line in pulmonary resections. Ann Thorac Surg 2001;71:319–23.

59. Oey IF, Jeyapalan K, Entwisle JJ, et al. Pseudo tumors of the lung after lung volume reduction surgery. Ann Thorac Surg 2004;77:1094–6.

60. Ahmed S, Marzouk KA, Bhuiya TA, et al. Asymptom-atic expectoration of surgical staples complicating lung volume reduction surgery. Chest 2001;119: 307–8.

61. Oey I, Waller DA. Metalloptysis: a late complication of lung volume reduction surgery. Ann Thorac Surg 2001;71:1694–5.

62. Shamji MF, Maziak DE, Shamji FM, et al. Surgical staple metalloptysis after apical bullectomy: a reac-tion to bovine pericardium? Ann Thorac Surg 2002; 74:258–61.

63. Provencher S, Deslauriers J. Late complication of bovine pericardium patches used for lung volume reduction surgery. Eur J Cardiothorac Surg 2003; 23:1059–61.

64. Iwasaki A, Yoshinaga Y, Shirakusa T. Successful removal of bovine pericardium by bronchoscope after lung volume reduction surgery. Ann Thorac Surg 2004;78:2156–7.

65. Fernandez E, Lopez de Castro PL, Tapia G, et al. Pseudotumor associated with polytetrafluoroethylene sleeves. Eur J Cardiothorac Surg 2008;33:937–8.

randomised controlled trial. J Cardiothorac Surg 2009;4:37–42.

# Postoperative Strategies to Treat Permanent Air Leaks

Federico Venuta, MD*, Erino A. Rendina, MD,
Tiziano De Giacomo, MD, Giorgio F. Coloni, MD

## KEYWORDS

- Air leaks • Lung resection • Pneumoperitoneum
- One-way valves • Pleurodesis • Lung volume reduction

Air leakage after pulmonary resections is considered the most prevalent postoperative problem, and it is often the only morbidity identified.[1,2] This common accident usually is not considered a complication per se but because it favors an increased rate of other complications and the duration and costs of hospitalization.[1,2] Air leaks are considered prolonged or persistent if they last for more than 5 to 7 days[3]; this happens in 8% to 26% of patients undergoing routine pulmonary resections.[1,4–7] When an air leak is still present on the fourth postoperative day, the chance of air leak on postoperative day 7 is 83%.[8]

Emphysema is clearly the primary risk factor both in the group of patients undergoing standard lobectomy[9] and, more obviously, among those undergoing lung volume reduction surgery (LVRS).[10] This basically is related to the anatomic modifications developed in this subset of patients, with continuous airway inflammation, fibroblasts derangement, and collagen production and healing impairment; continuous steroid administration contributes to the former aspect. Although chronic obstructive pulmonary disease (COPD) is the leading risk factor, there are other preoperative and intraoperative predictive variables that might contribute to the development of persistent air leaks: age, infections, associated parenchymal (interstitial) disease, diabetes mellitus, administration of induction therapy, malnutrition, tissue hypoxia, presence of adhesions or incomplete fissures, upper lobectomy or bilobectomy.[11] The incidence of this problem is similar in patients undergoing open and thoracoscopic procedures.

Ideally, treatment begins with prevention; patients should be well prepared before surgery. Also, intraoperative strategies to prevent and manage air leaks and residual spaces should be attempted.

Once an air leak develops, in most of the cases it will seal spontaneously within 2 or 3 days of operation.[2] When it persists longer, parenchymal leakage (alveolar–pleural fistula) should be distinguished immediately from bronchopleural fistulas; the latter poses serious problems and requires different treatment strategies including early reoperation, closure, and protection of the suture line with well vascularized flaps.

The underlying mechanisms of spontaneous air leak resolution are still unknown, although the development of pleural–pleural adhesions seems the most plausible. This mechanism could be postulated since in patients without pleural apposition (presence of persistent air space) the leakage usually last longer, and management is a much more formidable problem.

The postoperative approach to a prolonged air leak includes management of the pleural drainage and residual space, pleurodesis, pneumoperitoneum, deployment of endobronchial one-way valves, and potential reoperation.

## PLEURAL DRAIN MANAGEMENT

Although most of the air leaks resolve spontaneously within the first 3 or 4 postoperative days, it is always difficult, if not impossible, to predict how long they will last and which will stop early.

Department of Thoracic Surgery, University of Rome SAPIENZA, V.le del Policlinico, 00161 Rome, Italy
* Corresponding author. Cattedra di Chirurgia Toracica, Policlinico Umberto I, Università di Roma SAPIENZA, V.le del Policlinico, 00161 Rome, Italy.
E-mail address: federico.venuta@uniroma1.it

Thorac Surg Clin 20 (2010) 391–397
doi:10.1016/j.thorsurg.2010.03.004
1547-4127/10/$ – see front matter © 2010 Elsevier Inc. All rights reserved.

The general practice with chest drainage is based upon the importance given to the assumption that achieving pleural apposition is the most important factor to help healing; it is generally believed that some level of suction favors apposition between the parietal and visceral pleura. Although there is no clear evidence to support this practice, most surgeons tend to place chest drains at –20 cm $H_2O$ suction after pulmonary resections; the tubes are generally converted to water seal only when the leakage is minimal or absent. However, the attempt to achieve pleural apposition should be balanced with the need to minimize air flow through the visceral pleura defect.

The experience with LVRS progressively stimulated surgeons to evaluate different algorithms to interrupt air leaks. In fact, it looks like in this high-risk population, the standard negative suction might contribute to prolong air leaks.[12,13] On the base of these observations, most surgeons started to use a reduced suction level (–10 cm $H_2O$) or water seal alone; this new policy appears to have significantly contributed to reducing the duration of the leakage and related morbidity. It also supports the theory that reducing the flow through the visceral pleura defect might play a predominant role. There are several randomized, nonrandomized, and retrospective studies in the non-LVRS population. Among five prospective randomized studies,[14–18] three found a benefit with early water seal; one reported no difference between water seal and suction, and one found water seal moderately detrimental. One of the studies[17] evaluated an alternative suction protocol with –10 cm $H_2O$ suction during the night and water seal during the day from postoperative day 1. The aim of the authors was to combine the advantages of suction and water seal: pleural apposition and reduction of air flow through visceral pleura defects; this approach would also simplify early ambulation. This protocol did not show any difference in the duration of air leak between the two groups; however, in the alternate suction group, there was a shorter duration of chest tube and hospital stay and fewer prolonged air leaks.

In these randomized studies, the groups performing chest radiograph after placement to water seal reported that approximately 25% of patients developed a significant pneumothorax requiring suction re-establishment; however, none of these pneumothoraces were clinically remarkable, and no patients had evident pleural effusions or residual air spaces. On the base of these studies it is extremely difficult to design an algorithm to direct postoperative management of pleural drains. One additional help might come from the new digitalized suction systems. In particular, the DigiVent electronic device (Millicore AB, Stockholm, Sweden) contributes to monitor air flow through the drain and also inspiratory and expiratory pleural pressures.[19,20]

This monitoring system showed that chest drainage suction decreases differential pleural pressure after upper lobectomy[21] and allowed the application of a protocol for chest tube removal featuring a continuous recording of air leaks. This protocol allowed a reduction of chest tube duration, hospital stay and costs.[22]

The vast majority of the studies indicate that in most patients undergoing lobectomy, segmentectomy, and wedge resections, reducing suction below the traditional –20 cm $H_2O$ may be of help, even while the leakage persists. However, the ideal algorithm remains to be defined.

In the era of cost containment, fast-tracking protocols have been developed to shorten the length of hospitalization after lobectomy.[23,24] The use of ambulatory one-way valves applied to the chest drainage has greatly facilitated this process.[5,25] These devices must be used with close outpatient follow-up.[25] Heimelich[26] developed this valve for chest drainage in 1968, and since then, this device has been increasingly used to allow early discharge, not only after standard lung resections, but also after LVRS.[25] Air leaks treated with this device seem to close faster than expected, although there are no objective data supporting this impression or even to understand the mechanism of action. Significant air leaks or incomplete lung expansion traditionally have been considered contraindications to the use of the Heimlich valve.[26–30] In the series reported by Mc Kenna and colleagues,[25] however, this device was used even if the air leak was large or if there was an apical air space as large as 7 cm. The use of this valve is also important from the psychological point of view, since most of these patients are prone to depression and anxiety mainly related to the trauma of surgery, the nature of their disease, and the potential urge to begin adjuvant treatment. With the Heimlich valve, outpatient ambulation and independence are greatly facilitated. Monitoring of air leaks in patients with this device requires careful judgment; there is often little or no leakage with tidal breathing, but the leak becomes evident with cough or forced exhalation. If a residual space is present, this may be the only source of faced leak. In these situations, a trial of provocative clamping, especially in LVRS patients, might be of help to allow safe tube removal.[5,31]

## PLEURODESIS

Although conservative treatment ("wait and see") often allows closure of the air leak within a reasonable time, sometimes a more aggressive approach may be required.

If the residual lung is fully expanded, pleurodesis might be a suitable option to facilitate sealing of the visceral pleura. Tetracycline, quinacrine, talcum, and silver nitrate have been employed successfully in selected cases.[32–36] All these chemical agents have been able to favor pleural inflammation with encouraging results; however, none contributed to definitively solve the problem in all patients.

Autologous pleural blood patch has been employed repeatedly.[37–40] This technique was first reported by Robinson,[37] who described an 85% success rate in a series of 25 patients receiving one to three instillations of 50 mL of blood through the chest tubes. These data subsequently were confirmed by other reports.[38,39] The sealing effect can be explained by the direct mechanical action of the fibrin produced by the patch and the inflammatory reaction resulting from the presence of blood in the pleural cavity. This might be the primary factor to induce adhesion between the visceral and parietal pleura layers. One of the points that still remain open is related to the amount of blood that should be instilled inside the chest to obtain positive results. The authors previously reported a prospective study[40] evaluating outcome after pleurodesis with two different amounts of autologous blood (50 mL vs 100 mL). Pleurodesis with 50 mL of blood was effective and allowed closure of postoperative air leaks in a short period of time; however, the instillation of 100 mL of blood increased effectiveness and allowed sealing in less than 24 hours in most of the patients. Careful sterile manipulation of the system during the procedure is mandatory to avoid infections. In the authors' series, there was no procedure-related morbidity; there was no tension within the chest due to blood clotting. Additionally, the chest tube was not occluded, having been flushed with 20 mL of normal saline to prevent this complication; this allowed the authors to avoid tension pneumothorax as experienced by others.[41] Other complications were reported previously by others: fever and colonization of the pleural fluid.[38]

The autologous blood patch pleurodesis, which can be included among common bedside procedures, is easy to perform, safe, effective, and it does not add costs. It could be used as a first-line early maneuver to help solving this common and unpleasant problem.

Glues and sealants are extensively used intraoperatively; however, they very rarely are employed during the postoperative course because of the impossibility to blindly direct the flow toward the air leak source. If a bronchopleural fistula is present at the level of the bronchial stump, however, their use has been described with encouraging results.[42]

The authors' group is gaining increasing experience with the use of autologous platelet–leukocyte gel,[43] especially when the air leak is associated with a residual pleural space infected or potentially infected. This is a relatively new technology for the stimulation and acceleration of soft tissue and bone healing.[44] The gel can be applied to a variety of tissues, where it releases a high concentration of platelet-growing factor that is able to enhance tissue healing. In addition, leukocytes provide antimicrobial activity that may contribute to prevent or treat local infection.[44–46] The platelet–leukocyte-enriched gel is prepared from freshly drawn autologous blood; it comprises a small volume of plasma with fibrinogen, platelets, and leukocytes. Platelets become immediately activated by the interaction with thrombin, which is the most powerful platelet activator; this forms a sticky platelets aggregate. Besides a high concentration of platelets, leukocytes are also present (the concentration is two to four times higher than in the whole blood), including neutrophilic granulocytes and monocytes that are extremely active against bacteria. Also, platelets contain numerous antimicrobial peptides that usually are released after activation.[46] This gel previously was used to treat chronic nonhealing wounds[47,48] and large bone defects.[49] It recently has been employed also to prevent sternal infections after cardiac surgery procedures.[50] In the authors' hands, this gel has been employed several times to stop alveolar leakage associated with infected pleural spaces persisting for more than 3 to 4 weeks after pulmonary resections notwithstanding numerous attempts with other techniques, including blood patch and failed reoperation.

## PNEUMOPERITONEUM

Pneumoperitoneum initially was described in patients with emphysema at the beginning of the past century by Reich.[51] In these patients, the consequent transitory elevation of the diaphragm was associated with a decrease of dyspnea. The procedure recently was rediscovered to treat prolonged air leaks, space problems, or both occurring after pulmonary resections.[52–56] Pneumoperitoneum can be performed both intraoperatively, if those problems can be anticipated, or postoperatively. One or two liters of air usually are injected in the peritoneal cavity. The procedure usually is employed after lower lobectomy or bilobectomy, and it is supposed to work by achieving visceral and parietal pleural apposition. The air under the diaphragm temporarily elevates it, allowing pleural adhesion; this air is absorbed slowly over the 7 to 14 following days. The diaphragm then slowly descends, bringing with it the remaining lung that is now stuck. This process helps to eliminate residual spaces located at the base of the chest and leakages. Differences in the degree of diaphragmatic elevation have been observed[55] from one patient to the other, despite the procedure having placed the same amount of air and removed the same amount of lung parenchyma. Diaphragmatic elevation is probably influenced by several variables, including compliance of the residual homolateral and contralateral lung, the diaphragm, the mediastinum, and the actual distribution of air after insufflation. Also, temporary catheters can be placed under the diaphragm and brought through the skin.[52] This allows air to be insufflated each day postoperatively to maintain upward diaphragmatic displacement. The authors also have reported that air leaks and pleural space problems are more difficult to treat with pneumoperitoneum among patients who have undergone induction chemotherapy.[56] Previous abdominal procedures are not an absolute contraindication, but they should be considered carefully. This technique also was employed to treat air leaks and spaces after LVRS.[52]

## ENDOBRONCHIAL ONE-WAY VALVES

The inability to find an effective strategy to prevent and treat postoperative air leaks and the considerable morbidity related to this problem have prompted the need for minimally invasive nonsurgical approaches.

Endobronchial one-way valves (Zephir EBV; previously Emphasys, Redwood City, CA, USA. Currently Pulmonx Incorporated Redwood City, CA, USA) initially were developed for bronchoscopic lung volume reduction (BLVR) in patients with emphysema. They can be deployed through the operative channel of the fiberoptic bronchoscope and are able to block inflow into targeted areas of the lung.[57,58] These valves are well tolerated and can be removed easily if required. Many reports on small series of patients address the use of this device in patients with prolonged air leaks,[59–63] but only one[64] includes a reasonable number of cases collected from 17 different

centers; however, out of 40 patients included in this study, only 7 had postoperative air leaks. Of these seven patients, three had continuous air leaks, and four had only expiratory leakage. The mean number of valves placed was 2.28 plus or minus 1.1. No follow-up specific for these seven patients is reported in the manuscript; however, out of the 40 patients enrolled in this study, 19 (47.5%) had complete resolution of the air leak; 18 (45%) had a reduction. Two had no change, and one had no reported outcome. The mean time from valve deployment to chest tube removal was 21 days, and from the procedure to hospital discharge, the mean time was 19 plus or minus 28 days. Eight patients had the valves eventually removed. On the base of these initial reports, the use on endobronchial one-way valves can be considered an effective second-line intervention for patients with prolonged pulmonary air leaks.

## REOPERATION

Surgical re-exploration is rare. In the National Emphysema Treatment Trial, only 2.9% of patients required such intervention.[10] This approach should be considered only when other more conservative options have been attempted without success. Waiting too long, however, might be self-defeating, since the main risk is the development of polymicrobial or fungal empyema. The indication for reoperation is based on the magnitude of the leakage, the duration, and, as previously reported, failure of previous attempts.

The choice of operation depends on whether a residual space is present and on the quality of the residual lung. Thoracoscopy or open procedures should be selected on a case-by-case basis, on the base of the personal skills of each surgeon and the previous approach. Bronchoscopy is crucial to rule out the presence of bronchopleural fistula. If the residual lung is relatively normal, the leak can be restapled or oversewn with excellent results. Pleurectomy or mechanical pleurodesis can be added to improve results when pleural apposition is achieved. At reoperation, the diaphragm can be transiently paralyzed to allow better pleural apposition. Topical sealants might be used. An anatomic lobectomy (if not previously performed) should be considered only in extreme situations.

If a residual pleural cavity remains in conjunction with a persistent air leak, the volume of the space should be reduced. Potential strategies include filling with muscle transposition,[65,66] omentum transposition,[67] thoracoplasty, and even the creation of an open window for packing.[68]

# REFERENCES

1. Abolhoda A, Liu D, Brooks A, et al. Prolonged air leak following radical upper lobectomy: an analysis of incidence and possible risk factors. Chest 1998; 113:1507–10.

2. Okereke I, Murthy SC, Alster JM, et al. Characterization and importance of air leak after lobectomy. Ann Thorac Surg 2005;79:1167–73.

3. Kirsh MM, Rotman H, Beherendt DM, et al. Complications of pulmonary resection. Ann Thorac Surg 1975;20:215–36.

4. Varela G, Jimenez MF, Novoa N, et al. Estimating hospital costs attributable to prolonged air leak in pulmonary lobectomy. Eur J Cardiothorac Surg 2005;27:329–33.

5. Cerfolio RJ, Bass CS, Pask AH, et al. Predictors and treatment of persistent air leaks. Ann Thorac Surg 2002;73:1727–30.

6. Irshad K, Feldman LS, Chu VF, et al. Causes of increased length of hospitalization on a general thoracic surgery service: a prospective observational study. Can J Surg 2002;45:264–8.

7. Bardell T, Petsikas D. What keeps postpulmonary resection patients in hospital? Can Respir J 2003; 10:86–9.

8. Cerfolio RJ, Tummala RP, Holman WL, et al. A prospective algorithm for the management of air leaks after pulmonary resection. Ann Thorac Surg 1998;66:1726–30.

9. Brunelli A, Monteverde M, Borri A, et al. Predictors of prolonged air leak after pulmonary lobectomy. Ann Thorac Surg 2004;77:1205–10.

10. DeCamp MM, Blackstone EH, Naunheim KS, et al. Patient and surgical factors influencing air leak after lung volume reduction surgery: lessons learned from the National Emphysema Treatment Trial. Ann Thorac Surg 2006;82:197–206.

11. Shrager JB, DeCamp MM, Murthy SC. Intraoperative and postoperative management of air leaks in patients with emphysema. Thorac Surg Clin 2009; 19:223–31.

12. Cooper JD, Patterson GA, Sundaresan RS, et al. Results of 150 consecutive bilateral lung volume reduction procedures in patients with severe emphysema. J Thorac Cardiovasc Surg 1996;112: 1319–29.

13. Cooper JD, Patterson GA. Lung volume reduction surgery for severe emphysema. Chest Surg Clin N Am 1995;5:815–31.

14. Cerfolio RJ, Bass C, Katholi CR. Prospective randomized trial compares suction versus water seal for air leaks. Ann Thorac Surg 2001;71: 1613–7.

15. Marshall MB, Deeb ME, Bleier JI, et al. Suction vs water seal after pulmonary resection: a randomized prospective study. Chest 2002;121:831–5.

16. Brunelli A, Monteverde M, Borri A, et al. Comparison of water seal and suction after pulmonary lobectomy: a prospective, randomized trial. Ann Thorac Surg 2004;77:1932–7.

17. Brunelli A, Sabbatini A, Xiume F, et al. Alternate suction reduces prolonged air leak after pulmonary lobectomy: a randomized comparison versus water seal. Ann Thorac Surg 2005;80: 1052–5.

18. Alphonso N, Tan C, Utley M, et al. A prospective randomized controlled trial of suction versus non-suction to the underwater seal drains following lung resection. Eur J Cardiothorac Surg 2005;27: 391–4.

19. Dernevick L, Belboul A, Radberg G. Initial experience with the world's first digital drainage system. The benefits of recording air leaks with graphic presentation. Eur J Cardiothorac Surg 2007;31: 209–13.

20. Varela G, Jimenez MF, Novoa NM, et al. Postoperative chest tube management: measuring air leak using and electronic device decreases variability in the clinical practice. Eur J Cardiothorac Surg 2009; 35:28–31.

21. Varela G, Brunelli A, Jimenez MF, et al. Chest drainage suction decreases differential pleural pressure after upper lobectomy and has no effect after lower lobectomy. Eur J Cardiothorac Surg 2010;37: 531–4.

22. Brunelli A, Salati M, Refai M, et al. Evaluation of a new chest tube removal protocol using digital air leak monitoring after lobectomy: a prospective randomized trial. Eur J Cardiothorac Surg 2010;37: 56–60.

23. McKenna RJ Jr, Mahtabifard A, Pickens A, et al. Fast-tracking after video-assisted thoracoscopic surgery lobectomy, segmentectomy and pneumonectomy. Ann Thorac Surg 2007;84:1663–7.

24. Bryant AS, Cerfolio RJ. The influence of preoperative risk stratification on fast tracking patients after pulmonary resections. Thorac Surg Clin 2008;18: 113–8.

25. McKenna RJ Jr, Fischel RJ, Brenner M, et al. Use of the Heimlich valve to shorten hospital stay after lung reduction surgery for emphysema. Ann Thorac Surg 1996;61:1115–7.

26. Heimlich HG. Valve drainage of the pleural cavity. Dis Chest 1968;53:282–6.

27. Cannon WB, Mark JBD, Jamplins RW. Pneumothorax: a therapeutic update. Am J Surg 1981;142: 26–9.

28. Schweitzer EJ, Hauer JM, Swan KG, et al. Use of the Heimlich valve in a compact autotrasfusion device. J Trauma 1987;27:537–42.

29. Driver AG, Peden JG, Adams HG, et al. Heimlich valve treatment of *Pneumocystis carinii* associated pneumothorax. Chest 1991;100:281–2.

30. Valee P, Sullivan M, Richardson H, et al. Sequential treatment of a simple pneumothorax. Ann Emerg Med 1988;17:936–42.

31. Kischner PA. Provocative clamping and removal of chest tubes despite persistent leak. Ann Thorac Surg 1992;53:740–1.

32. Almassi GH, Haasler GB. Chemical pleurodesis in the presence of persistent air leak. Ann Thorac Surg 1989;47:786–7.

33. Checani V. Tetracycline pleurodesis for persistent air leak. Ann Thorac Surg 1990;49:166–7.

34. Janzing HM, Derom A, Derom E, et al. Intrapleural quinacrine instillation for recurrent pneumothorax or persistent air leak. Ann Thorac Surg 1993;55:368–71.

35. Baumann MH, Strange C. The clinician's perspective on pneumothorax management. Chest 1997;112:822–88.

36. Gallivan GJ. Pleurodesis and silver nitrate. Chest 2001;119:1624.

37. Robinson CL. Autologous blood for pleurodesis in recurrent and chronic spontaneous pneumothorax. Can J Surg 1987;30:428–9.

38. Lang–Lazduski L, Coonar AS. A prospective study of autologous blood patch pleurodesis for persistent air leak after pulmonary resection. Eur J Cardiothorac Surg 2004;26:897–900.

39. Rivas de Andres JJ, Blanco S, de la Torre M. Post-surgical pleurodesis with autologous blood in patients with persistent air leak. Ann Thorac Surg 2000;70:270–2.

40. Andreetti C, Venuta F, Anile M, et al. Pleurodesis with an autologous blood patch to prevent persistent air leaks after lobectomy. J Thorac Cardiovasc Surg 2007;133:759–62.

41. Williams P, Lang R. Tension pneumothorax complicating autologous "blood patch" pleurodesis. Thorax 2005;60:1066–7.

42. Shimizu J, Takizawa M, Yachi T, et al. Postoperative bronchial stump fistula responding well to occlusion with metallic coils and fibrin glue via a tracheostomy. Ann Thorac Cardiovasc Surg 2005;11:104–8.

43. De Giacomo T, Diso D, Ferrazza G, et al. Successful treatment of infected residual pleural space after pulmonary resection with autologous platelet – leukocyte gel. Ann Thorac Surg 2009;88:1689–91.

44. Everts PA, Overdevest EP, Jakimovicz JJ. The use of autologous platelet–leukocyte gels to enhance the healing process in surgery. Surg Endosc 2007;21:2063–8.

45. Wareham EE, Barber H, McGoey JS, et al. The persistent pleural space following partial pulmonary resection. J Thorac Surg 1956;31:593–9.

46. Krijgsveld J, Zaat SA, Meeldijk J, et al. Thrombocidins, microbicidal proteins from human blood platelets, are C – terminal deletion products of CXC chemokines. J Biol Chem 2000;275:20374–81.

47. Mazzucco L, Medici D, Serra M, et al. The use of autologous platelet gel to treat difficult-to-heal wounds: a pilot study. Transfusion 2004;44:1013–8.

48. Henderson JL, Cupp CL, Ross EV, et al. The effects of autologous platelet gel on wound healing. Ear Nose Throat J 2003;82:598–602.

49. Smrke D, Gubina B, Domanovic D, et al. Allogenic platelet gel with autologous cancellous bone graft for the treatment of a large bone defect. Eur Surg Res 2007;39:170–4.

50. Trowbridge CC, Stammers AH, Woods E, et al. Use of platelet gel and its effects on infection in cardiac surgery. J Extra Corpor Technol 2005;37:381–6.

51. Reich L. Der Einfluss des Pneumoperitoneum auf das Lungen—Emphysema. Wien Arch Finn Med 1924;8:245–60 [in German].

52. Handy JR, Judson MA, Zeliner JL. Pneumoperitoneum to treat air leaks and spaces after lung volume reduction operations. Ann Thorac Surg 1997;64:1803–5.

53. Yusen RD, Littenberg B. Technology assessment and pneumoperitoneum therapy for air leaks and pleural spaces. Ann Thorac Surg 1997;64:1583–4.

54. Carbognani P, Spaggiari L, Solli P, et al. Pneumoperitoneum for prolonged air leaks after lower lobectomies. Ann Thorac Surg 1998;66:604–5.

55. Cerfolio RJ, Holman WL, Katholi CR. Pneumoperitoneum after concomitant resection of the right middle and lower lobes (bilobectomy). Ann Thorac Surg 2000;70:942–7.

56. De Giacomo T, Rendina EA, Venuta F, et al. Pneumoperitoneum for the management of pleural space problems associated with major pulmonary resections. Ann Thorac Surg 2001;72:1716–9.

57. Venuta F, Rendina EA, De Giacomo T, et al. Bronchoscopic procedures for emphysema treatment. Eur J Cardiothorac Surg 2006;29:281–7.

58. Venuta F, De Giacomo T, Rendina EA, et al. Bronchoscopic lung volume reduction with one way valves in patients with heterogeneous emphysema. Ann Thorac Surg 2005;79:411–6.

59. Fann JI, Berry GJ, Burdon TA. The use of endobronchial valve device to eliminate air leak. Respir Med 2006;100:1402–6.

60. De Giacomo T, Venuta F, Diso D, et al. Successful treatment with one way endobronchial valve of large air leakage complicating narrow bore enteral feeding tube malposition. Eur J Cardiothorac Surg 2006;30:811–2.

61. Snell GI, Holsworth L, Fowler S, et al. Occlusion of a bronchocutaneous fistula with endobronchial one way valves. Ann Thorac Surg 2005;80:1930–2.

62. Anile M, Venuta F, De Giacomo T, et al. Treatment of persistent air leakage with endobronchial one way valves. J Thorac Cardiovasc Surg 2006;132:711–2.

63. Toma TP, Kon OM, Oldfield W, et al. Reduction of persistent air leak with endoscopic valve implants. Thorax 2007;62:830–3.
64. Travaline JM, McKenna RJ Jr, De Giacomo T, et al. Treatment of persistent pulmonary air leaks using endobronchial valves. Chest 2009;136:355–60.
65. Colwell AS, Mentzer SJ, Vargas SO, et al. The role of muscle flaps in pulmonary aspergillosis. Plast Reconstr Surg 2003;111:1147–50.
66. Francel TJ, Lee GW, Mackinnon SE, et al. Treatment of long standing tracheostoma and bronchopleural fistula without pulmonary resection in high risk patients. Plast Reconstr Surg 1997;99:1046–53.
67. Nonami Y, Ogoshi S. Omentopexy for empyema due to lung fistula following lobectomy. A case report. J Cardiovasc Surg (Torino) 1998;39:695–6.
68. Murthy SC. Air leak and pleural space management. Thorac Surg Clin 2006;16:261–5.

# The Management of Chest Tubes After Pulmonary Resection

Robert J. Cerfolio, MD, FCCP, Ayesha S. Bryant, MSPH, MD*

**KEYWORDS**

• Chest tube • Air leak • Pulmonary resection • Water seal

## HISTORY OF CHEST TUBES

Drainage of the space between the ribs and the lung, the pleural space, has been practiced since the time of Hippocrates.[1,2] He describes the use of an incision, cautery, and metal rods to remove "evil humors" from patients with a variety of poorly understood illnesses. Hunter, in 1800, used needle drainage to remove fluid from the pleural space, and in 1872, Playfair first placed a chest tube to underwater seal, similar to what is used today.[3,4] Gotthard Bülau, however, is credited as the originator of the first closed water seal drainage system. The improved outcome of using a closed system over the more popular open drainage system (ie, rib resection with open drainage or Eloesser flap) is derived from data accumulated by the US Army, which reported extensive experience from the battlefield and elsewhere. The mortality rate for empyema treated with rib resection and leaving the chest open compared with closed pleural drainage was 28% compared with 4%, respectively. Thus, closed pleural space drainage became the standard of care in the early twentieth century. The concept of underwater seal was born. In 1917, Evert Graham[5] described closed drainage for influenza empyema after a significant number of patients died after open drainage technique. Lilienthal,[6] in 1922, first used and later reintroduced closed pleural drainage in the postoperative care of patients after routine thoracic surgery.

Chest tubes have been given a variety of names over the years, including Bülau drains, intercostal catheters, and thoracostomy tubes. Whatever they are called, their function has been the same for more than 3000 years, to drain fluid or air from the pleural space. Modifications of the material used to make chest tubes themselves as well as to the pleural drainage systems have continued. Not only has the chest tube itself undergone improvements but also the drainage systems used have seen many modifications and improvements, including an air leak meter, smaller and more compact size to allow home discharge, and recently some feature digital measurements of air leaks as well as the digital record of the amount of effluent each hour.

## DEFINITION OF IMPORTANT TERMS

Before reviewing the data on chest tube management, several terms must be defined. There remains significant confusing about much of the vocabulary that is used for chests tubes and the pleural space. Although thoracic surgeons are the best-trained physicians to manage chest tubes and pleural space problems, they often do not speak the same language or recommend similar treatment algorithms even to each other. This

RJ Cerfolio was a speaker for E Plus Healthcare (PET scanners); speaker and consultant for Ethicon; consultant for NeoMend; speaker and consultant for Millicore (digital air leak device); speaker and consultant for Medela (digital air leak device); speaker for Teleflex (pleural drainage system); consultant for Closure Medical/Johnson & Johnson; speaker for OSI Pharmaceuticals; consultant and speaker for Atrium (drainage system); speaker for Oncotech (tumor markers); speaker for Covidien (staplers); and lecturer for Precision Therapeutics (tumor analysis of cancers).
Division of Cardiothoracic Surgery, University of Alabama at Birmingham, 703 19th Street South, ZRB 739, Birmingham, AL 35294, USA
* Corresponding author.
E-mail address: abryant@uab.edu

Thorac Surg Clin 20 (2010) 399–405
doi:10.1016/j.thorsurg.2010.04.001
1547-4127/10/$ – see front matter © 2010 Elsevier Inc. All rights reserved.

leads to confusion. Moreover, confidence in recommendations is eroded if they change with each surgeon who is on call.

The pleural space has a negative intrathoracic pressure and anything that disturbs this can lead to physiologic compromise. For this reason the first drainage systems featured a 3-bottle system (**Fig. 1**). A 1-bottle system was used initially; however, as the fluid or blood that drained from patients rose in the only bottle, it increased the resistance to further drainage. Moreover, the mixture of air in the bottle and blood from patients caused a foamy effluent to build up in the bottle, again impeding drainage. Therefore, a 2-bottle system quickly became adopted. The second bottle allowed fluid to drain into the first bottle only and the air escaped into the second. This prevented the foam from forming and the 2-bottle system had to be drained less frequently. The problem with the 2-bottle system was that the added length of the tubing increased the dead space and again added significant resistance. Some patients actually had reversal of flow and often their chest tube effluent would start to go back up into the tube and back into the pleural space of these patients. For that reason the famed 3-bottle system arrived (see **Fig. 1**). The third bottle allows for active suction to be exerted on the system. This active suction prevents the chest tube effluent from going back toward the patient. Essentially, all commercial systems use this technology now and some have a 1-way tip over valve.

## ACTIVE SUCTION COMPARED WITH PASSIVE SUCTION

An important distinction should be made between active suction and passive suction. Underwater seal or passive suction occurs when a chest tube is attached to a drainage system but there is no further suction added (most commonly from external tubes connected to the wall). This is often called a water seal because the tube is connected to a system that essentially has the distal end of the chest tube submerged under approximately 2 cm of water. During expiration or coughing, air from the pleural space is expelled through the tubing and overcomes the hydrostatic pressure. It also produces a siphon effect, which enhances drainage. This is why air leaks can be visualized in the water chamber in many commercial systems. Some feature an air leak meter to quantify the size of the air leak, ranging from 1 to 7.

When external suction is applied to the drainage system, this added suction is called active suction because it is added to the passive suction that already exists in the drainage system's underwater seal. Some refer to this as wall suction but new digital units are able to exert active suction on their own and do not require any wall suction attachments.

Once it was observed that a 3-bottle system clinically was best, companies began to come up with ways to add all 3 bottles into one compact, user-friendly, commercial system. Initially the suction that was added was termed, *wet suction*. The term, *wet*, was used because the suction had to be under water. These systems are safe, because it is difficult to exert greater than a $-15$ or $-20$ cm $H_2O$ pressure and they allowed inadequate airflow in patients who had a large air leak. In these systems, a certain level of water was needed and the amount of suction was determined by the height of water.

These wet systems have been replaced for the most part by dry suction for several reasons. In

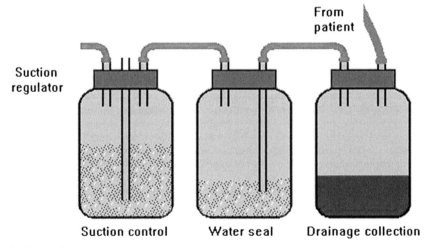

**Fig. 1.** 3-Bottle chest tube drainage system.

the wet systems, a continuous bubbling of suction under water was needed, which was was loud and annoying to patients and nurses. In addition, because the water was constantly evaporating, it had to be replaced, leading to an inconsistent amount of suction. Dry suction systems are easier to set up, provide higher levels of suction if needed, and are quieter. Probably most importantly, because they regulate the amount of suction not by a height or column of water but rather via a self-compensating regulator, they provide a more consistent amount of suction.[7] A final term needs to be addressed: a *fixed pleural space deficit* is defined as a nonresolving pneumothorax when the lung is fully expanded.[8]

## INITIAL EVALUATION OF AN AIR LEAK—IS IT REAL?

If confronted with an alveolar-pleural fistula (air leak), the clinician at the bedside must ensure that the leak is really from the patient and is not a system leak. All connections between the chest tube and the drainage system should be checked. When the leak is confirmed as coming from inside the patient's chest and not the system, it should be classified. Careful observation at the bedside reveals that the natural history of air leaks is based on two main features, the type of air leak (the qualitative aspect of the system, determined by when the air leak occurs during the respiratory cycle) and the size of the air leak (the quantitative aspect of the classification system). The authors have developed[9] and refined a classification[10] system for alveolar-pleural fistulas (air leaks), the Robert David Cerfolio Classification System for Air Leaks (RDC System), named after the first author's father. It is described at length elsewhere.[11] The authors believe that in the future, digital systems, already on the market, will replace this analog system. The full implementation of these systems, however, will be based on cost, and many hospitals outside of North America and Eastern Europe will probably continue to use the analog systems for several years.

## EVIDENCE-BASED MEDICINE FOR THE MANAGEMENT OF CHEST TUBES AFTER PULMONARY RESECTION

Over the past several years there has been an interest in bring the scientific method to chest tube management. A PubMed literature search shows that before 1996, there were fewer than 10 articles that described studies on how to manage air leaks and chest tubes. From 1997 to 2009, however, there were 11 publications by the authors (University of Alabama at Birmingham [UAB], Birmingham, AL, USA) and 9 from Brunelli (Umberto, Regional Hospital Ancona, Italy) on the management of chest tubes and air leaks. Therefore, many of the recommendation come from these two centers.

The study of the management of chest tubes is based on two factors that slow or prevent removal: air leaks and a high volume of pleural drainage. These two factors need to be considered separately and a more aggressive management style is needed to help speed the safe removal of chest tubes to decrease pain and to prevent empyema. Postoperative pain reduction improves respiratory mechanics and limits splinting and shallow breathing, thus reducing the chance for postoperative pneumonia and other complications.

## AIR LEAK MANAGEMENT

Air leaks are the most common complication after pulmonary resection. Historically, chest tubes were placed to suction after chest surgery to promote the drainage of fluids out of the chest. Because of this initial practice, wall suction or active suction (discussed previously) has been the historical and preferred setting for chest tubes. In 1996, the authors made the simple observation at the bedside that suction made air leaks bigger, thus theorizing that if the pleural-pleural apposition were maintained when chest tubes were placed to water seal (ie, there was no new pneumothorax) that a water seal helped air leaks stop sooner.

The authors and Brunelli and colleagues have studied the problem of alveolar-pleural fistulas (air leaks) using prospective randomized trials or predetermined algorithms in an attempt to bring some science to what had been a subjective art form. **Table 1** provides an overview of some of the larger prospective studies addressing the issue of chest tube management—placing chest tubes to water seal (passive suction) or to suction (active suction). Although overall review of this data leads to the conclusion that the optimal chest tube setting is not yet proved for all patients, certain definitive statements can be made from these reports.

The first prospective study, which was from the authors' group, found that most air leaks occurred during expiration.[9] Also reported in that first study was that pulmonary function testing consistent with emphysema increased the risk of having an air leak after pulmonary resection. This study showed that placing chest tubes on water seal not only was safe for air leaks but also seemed superior to suction at stopping leaks in patients who maintained parietal-pleural to visceral pleural

**Table 1**
**Recent studies evaluating the management of chest tubes in post-thoracotomy patients**

| Author, Year of Publication | Study Type | Comparison | Findings |
|---|---|---|---|
| Cerfolio et al,[10] 2001 | Prospective randomized trial (postpulmonary resection) | Suction POD 1, then randomized to S versus W on POD 2 | Water seal superior after POD 0 of suction |
| Marshall et al,[12] 2002 | Prospective randomized study (postpulmonary resection) | Initially S, then randomized to S or W | Water seal shorted the duration of AL and CT duration |
| Ayed,[13] 2003 | Prospective randomized (patients with spontaneous ptx) | S versus W | Water seal after brief period of suction decreased CT duration |
| Brunelli et al,[14] 2005 | Prospective randomized trial (postlobectomy with air leak on POD 1) | S versus W | No difference |
| Brunelli et al,[15] 2004 | Prospective randomized (postlobectomy) | Alternating S versus W | Alternating suction superior to water seal (reduced incidence of AL, decreased CT duration, LOS) |
| Cerfolio et al,[16] 2005 | Retrospective review (patients with ptx and air leak) | S versus W | Water seal superior unless ptx is large/symptomatic or patient develops subcutaneous emphysema |
| Okamoto et al,[17] 2006 | Retrospective | S versus W | No difference |

*Abbreviations:* AL, air leak; CT, chest tube; LOS, length of stay; POD, postoperative day; ptx, pneumothorax; S, suction; W, water seal.

apposition. It provided safety data to perform a prospective randomized study.

The second study on air leaks was also from the authors' institution at UAB. It was a prospective randomized trial of 140 patients, 33 of whom had air leaks.[10] This study showed that patients who had their tubes placed on water seal (passive suction) instead of wall suction (active suction) were more likely to have their leak stop. A water seal also made air leaks smaller. A water seal did not stop large expiratory leaks, however, because patients when placed to passive suction often developed a pneumothorax. The RDC system for air leaks was further refined and validated between blinded observers. The classification system has become a critical component for the management of tubes. It helps guide treatment. For example, if patients have an expiratory 5 leak, their tubes are best left on suction and not placed to water seal because an enlarging pneumothorax is probable. The passive suction (water seal) not stopping

these leaks corroborates one of Brunelli's theories. This may be because these leaks, when placed on water seal or passive suction, led to a pneumothorax. They are too large for passive suction and air is not fully evacuated from the pleural space. This prevented pleural-pleural apposition, thus the leak did not seal. This concept is supported by Brunelli and colleagues,[14] who favor active suction at night and passive suction during the day. This conclusion is from their 2005 study. They performed a randomized controlled trial comparing water seal (passive suction) to alternating wall suction (active suction) with water seal (passive suction) in postpulmonary resection patients. They used suction at night and waters seal during the day for ease of ambulation. They found that alternating suction with water seal was superior to water seal alone. Patients on the alternating treatments had a significantly shorter hospital length of stay and chest tube duration.[14] The authors believe this regimen may be best for a bigger air leak (>an expiratory 3) in many patients.

Marshall and colleagues[12] from The University of Pennsylvania reported another prospective randomized study and found that placing chest tubes on water seal (passive suction) after pulmonary resection shortens the duration of air leaks and decreases the time chest tubes remain in place. Brunelli and colleagues,[15] however, recently published a report on series of selected patients, many of whom had undergone pleural tenting. The investigators reported that those patients on water seal had more complications compared with those who were treated with suction. This finding needs to be further explored.

Other reports have found that if patients have large (E6 or E7) air leaks on postoperative day 1, they continue to have an air leak by postoperative day 4 irrespective of the chest tube management. These patients are discharged home (if otherwise ready for discharge) on a Heimlich valve.[18] Because of the accuracy and reliability of the classification system, these patients can be informed about the need for discharge with an indwelling tube early in their hospital course. This allows patients, families, nurses, and physicians to prepare mentally and physically for discharge home on a Heimlich valve. Moreover, this information has helped the authors care for patients with spontaneous pneumothoraces. If patients suffer their first spontaneous pneumothorax, the authors usually place a chest tube only and observe the patients. But if the air leak is large, an E4 or greater, the natural history of that leak is prolonged. The authors' most recent article on leaks reports that water seal is safe for patients with an air leak and a pneumothorax.[16] If the leak is large (>an E4) or the pneumothorax is large (>8 cm on a measurement scale defined in that article), however, the seal is not safe.

Another important aspect of air leak management is the use of intraoperative techniques to stop leaks. There are many studies that have evaluated the efficacy of using pulmonary sealants to prevent leaks.[19–21] There is only one Food and Drug Administration–approved pulmonary sealant and it is just coming to the market in 2010. Studies are under way to assess its efficacy and cost savings.

## TREATMENT OF PERSISTENT AIR LEAKS

The Society of Thoracic Surgeons' database defines persistent air leak as one that lasts more than 5 days. In the authors' practice, however, a persistent air leak is defined as one that prolongs hospitalization. If, on the third postoperative day,

the leak is larger than an forced expiratory 3 (FE3), it will not seal overnight. For that reason the patient's chest tubes are connected to a Heimlich valve or to an outpatient device (the authors have used Express [Atrium, Hudson, NH, USA], MINI Sahara [Teleflex, Research Triangle Park, NC, USA], and, most recently, Thopaz [Medela, Baar, Switzerland]). If a Heimlich valve is used, the other end is connected to a urinary leg bag or a compact portable drainage system. A chest x-ray (CXR) is obtained after 24 hours on the Heimlich valve, and if no new subcutaneous emphysema or no new or enlarging pneumothorax is seen, patients are discharged home on postoperative day 4 or 5. Neither a pneumothorax nor subcutaneous emphysema usually occurs unless the air leak is large, greater than an E4 in the RDC system. If a CXR identifies a problem, such as subcutaneous air or a new or enlarging pneumothorax, patients must be returned to water seal or $-10$ cm $H_2O$ of suction, whichever is needed to alleviate the pneumothorax. This process is repeated in 2 days. If a second pneumothorax occurs, the options are to perform a bedside chemical pleurodesis or to wait 48 hours. If a bedside pleurodesis is performed using doxycycline, the tubing cannot be clamped. Tubing should be hung well over a patient's bed so that after the sclerotic agent is shot into the tube, it is hung over the patient and then attached to the drainage system, which is placed on passive suction (water seal). Often, an extra length of rubber tubing is needed to accomplish this height. This technique allows the sclerotic agent to stay in the chest but air can escape.

## OUTPATIENT MANAGEMENT OF CHEST TUBES

Once patients are discharged home on an outpatient device, no specific instructions are needed. The authors use a daily subtherapeutic dose of cephalexin hydrochloride (Keflex, MiddleBrook Pharmaceuticals, West Lake, TX, USA) (500 mg once a day) as a prophylaxis measure to help prevent empyema and have shown this is safe and effective and that the chest tube can be removed in 2 weeks almost without exception even if patients still have a leak.[22] This is an important concept because many continue to have reservation about tube removal in patients with an air leak. Provocative chest tube clamping can be performed (described previously) if the leak is worrisome. More recently, the authors have switched from the Heimlich valve system to a compact, self-contained devise and have had success with this system because it allows better capturing of the effluent and is more compact, clean, and user friendly than the Heimlich valve hooked to a Foley catheter drainage bag.

## HIGH-VOLUME DRAINAGE

Although air leaks are the most common complication after pulmonary resection, it is the drainage of over 250 mL/day that is the most common cause of delayed discharged and chest tube removal in the United States. Many surgeons use this unproved strict criteria for the amount of drainage a tube can have before removing it. Patients often have chest tubes left in because the drainage was "greater than 150 mL/day," "greater than 50 mL/shift," or greater than "250 mL/day." Because this number seemed arbitrary and completely unsubstantiated by data, the authors performed a study in 2008[23] assessing the safety of the removal of tubes with higher outputs. In this study, the authors removed chest tubes when the drainage was 450 mL/day or less, if there was no air leak, and if cerebrospinal fluid (CSF), chylothorax, or hemothorax was ruled out. It seemed not only was the amount of drainage important but also the character of the drainage should be factor. If the effluent was clear and not CSF, blood, or chlye, then removal of the tube even with high drainage should be safe. This study included 2077 patients and only 11 (<1%) were readmitted for recurrent effusions. The authors concluded that chest tubes can be safely removed with up to 450 mL/day of nonchylous drainage after pulmonary resection, and higher numbers need to be tested because 450 mL is also arbitrary.

## THE ROLE OF DAILY CXRS

A final word about the use of daily CXRs is needed. Although the vast majority of surgeons ordered a daily CXR on patients with a chest tube in place, there are few data that show this is needed. CXRs are expensive and if done early in the morning, so as to be available for morning rounds, are disruptive and uncomfortable for patients. In the majority of patients, if postoperative recovery room film shows pleural-pleural apposition and patients do not develop an air leak or other clinical problems, daily CXRs rarely influence chest tube management or patient care decisions. If patients develop any type of clinical scenario that includes shortness of breath, decreasing saturation, or subcutaneous emphysema, then a film is needed and should be ordered.

In conclusion, air leaks are a common clinical problem after pulmonary resection. The management of tubes, drains, and air leak can be studied with randomized trials and objective data. A validated, objective classification system is now available and helps guide treatment, and new digital systems show great promise. Randomized studies have shown that placing chest tubes to water seal (passive suction) is superior to suction and better at stopping air leaks when a pneumothorax does not occur when patients are placed to water seal. Large leaks (ie, >E4), however, will probably fail water seal and patients may develop a pneumothorax or enlarging subcutaneous emphysema. In these patients or in others who lose pleural-pleural apposition on water seal (passive suction), some suction is best, and the Brunelli concept of alternating active suction at night with passive suction during the day is probably best. Prolonged air leaks are more common in patients with emphysematous lungs and with pulmonary resections that remove large amounts of lung. A pneumothorax itself is not an indication for suction because many patients have a fixed pleural space deficit. Finally, patients can safely go home with an air leak and with chest tubes in place. The tubes can be managed on an outpatient basis and then removed by postoperative day 21, even if patients still have an air leak as long as there is no subcutaneous emphysema or a symptomatic pneumothorax. Further randomized studies are needed.

## REFERENCES

1. Chadwich J, Mann WH. The medical works of Hippocrates. Springfield: Charles C Thomas; 1950.
2. Miller KS, Sahn SA. Chest tubes. Indications, technique management and complications. Chest 1987;91:258–64.
3. Hochberg LA. Thoracic surgery before the 20th century. New York: Vantage Press; 1960. p. 244.
4. Bowditch HI. On pleuritic effusions and the necessity of paracentesis for their removal. Am J Med Sci 1852;22:320.
5. Graham EA. Some fundamental considerations in the treatment of empyema thoracis. St Louis: Mosby; 1925. p. 7–110.
6. Lilienthal H. Pulmonary resection for bronchiectasis. Ann Surg 1922;75:257.
7. Cerfolio RJ. Closed drainage and suction systems. Pearson's Thoracic and Esophageal Surgery. 3rd editon. Philadelphia: Churchill, Livingstone; 2008. p. 1147–63.
8. Cerfolio RJ. Recent advances in the treatment of air leaks. Curr Opin Pulm Med 2005;11:319–24.
9. Cerfolio RJ, Tummala RP, Holman WL, et al. A prospective algorithm for the management of air

leaks after pulmonary resection. Ann Thorac Surg 1998;66:1726–31.

10. Cerfolio RJ, Bass CS, Katholi CR, et al. Prospective randomized trial compares suction versus water seal for air leaks. Ann Thorac Surg 2001;71:1613–7.

11. Cerfolio RJ. Advances in thoracostomy tube management. Surg Clin North Am 2002;82:833–48.

12. Marshall MB, Deeb ME, Bleier JI, et al. Suction vs water seal after pulmonary resection: a randomized prospective study. Chest 2002;121:831–5.

13. Ayed AK. Suction versus water seal after thoracoscopy for primary spontaneous pneumothorax: prospective randomized study. Ann Thorac Surg 2003;75:1593–6.

14. Brunelli A, Sabbatini A, Xiume F, et al. Alternate suction reduces prolonged air leak after pulmonary lobectomy: a randomized comparison versus water seal. Ann Thorac Surg 2005;80:1052–5.

15. Brunelli A, Monteverde M, Borri A, et al. Comparison of water seal and suction after pulmonary lobectomy: a prospective, randomized trial. Ann Thorac Surg 2004;77:1932–7.

16. Cerfolio RJ, Bryant AS, Singh S, et al. The management of chest tubes in patients with a pneumothoerax and an air leak after pulmonary resection. Chest 2005;128:816.

17. Okamoto OJ, Fukuyama Y, Ushijima C, et al. The use of waters seal to manage air leaks after a pulmonary lobectomy: a retrospective study. Ann Thorac Cardiovasc Surg 2006;12:242–4.

18. Heimlich HJ. Valve drainage of the pleural cavity. Dis Chest 1986;53:282–7.

19. Lang G, Csekeo A, Stamatis G, et al. Efficacy and safety of topical application of human fibrinogen/thrombin-coated collagen patch for treatment of air leakage after standard lobectomy. Eur J Cardiothorac Surg 2004;25:160–6.

20. Porte HL, Jany T, Akkad R, et al. Randomized controlled trial of a synthetic sealant for preventing air leaks after lobectomy. Ann Thorac Surg 2001; 71:1618–22.

21. Wain JC, Kaiser LR, Johnsotne DW, et al. Trial of a novel synthetic sealant in preventing air leaks after lung resection. Ann Thorac Surg 2001;71: 1623–9.

22. Cerfolio RJ, Minnich DJ, Bryant AS. The removal of chest tubes despite an air leak or a pneumothorax. Ann Thorac Surg 2009;87:1690–4.

23. Cerfolio RJ, Bryant AS. Results of a prospective algorithm to remove chest tubes after pulmonary resection with high output. J Thorac Cardiovasc Surg 2008;135:269–73.

# The Cost of Air Leak: Physicians' and Patients' Perspectives

Adam Lackey, MD[a], John D. Mitchell, MD[b],*

**KEYWORDS**
- Air leak • Postoperative complication
- Cost • Pulmonary resection

Despite ongoing technical advances and refinements in surgical technique, the occurrence of a prolonged parenchymal air leak (PAL) after pulmonary resection remains an all too frequent complication. Traditionally depicted as an air leak persisting beyond 7 days, perhaps the best definition of a prolonged leak is one that delays hospital discharge; in the modern surgical era, this may be classified as an air leak persisting beyond 5 days.[1,2] The incidence of PAL varies in the literature from 5% to 25%,[1–7] and is heavily influenced by the presence of underlying lung disease[7–9] and the type of lung resection performed.[3,5,10] For example, in the National Emphysema Treatment Trial, the incidence of prolonged air leak following lung volume reduction surgery (LVRS) was approximately 50%, with 12% of subjects having a persistent leak at 30 days.[9] Efforts to reduce the incidence of PAL using preventative measures have been inconsistent at best.[9,11]

The impact, or cost, of a complication such as prolonged air leak differs for patients and the involved health care providers. In both cases, the cost is in part determined by the treatment strategy chosen to deal with the complication. In this article, the authors explore the impact of a PAL from the perspective of physicians and patients, including factors common to both groups.

## FINANCIAL COSTS

The presence of a prolonged air leak increases length of stay (LOS),[2,3,5,10,12,13] and as a result, the hospital costs associated with the procedure. In a study designed to estimate hospital costs associated with PAL, Varela and colleagues[2] described 238 subjects undergoing pulmonary lobectomy over a 3-year period, noting PAL in 23 subjects (9.7%). Subjects remained hospitalized until cessation of the leak, allowing for chest tube removal. As a result, the mean LOS for subjects with a PAL was twice that noted for the non-PAL cases. The total additional hospital costs attributed to persistent air leak was calculated to be 39,437 €, or roughly $53,000 (using exchange rate at the time of publication).

The excess hospital costs noted in the Varela and colleagues[2] study resulted exclusively from the additional inpatient days and pharmacy charges incurred by the subjects with PAL until the leak resolved. It is rare that a second surgical procedure is needed to address the (parenchymal-based) leak; in almost all cases, expectant management is successful. However, the presence of air leak after pulmonary resection, particularly if prolonged, has been associated with an increased incidence of other postoperative complications.[2,10,14] These complications, such as atelectasis, retained secretions, and empyema, may require additional treatment leading to increased hospital costs. Depending on interpretation, these costs may prove problematic in a capitated reimbursement system. The Centers for Medicare and Medicaid Services[15] has recently initiated a program denying payment for inpatient services derived

[a] Department of Surgery, University of Colorado Denver School of Medicine, 12631 East 17th Avenue, C-302, Aurora, CO 80045, USA
[b] General Thoracic Surgery, Division of Cardiothoracic Surgery, University of Colorado Denver School of Medicine, 12631 East 17th Avenue, C-310, Aurora, CO 80045, USA
* Corresponding author.
E-mail address: john.mitchell@ucdenver.edu

Thorac Surg Clin 20 (2010) 407–411
doi:10.1016/j.thorsurg.2010.04.004

from treatment for "potentially preventable complications."[16] Examples of such complications include line sepsis, pressure ulcers, air embolism, patient falls, and mediastinitis after cardiac surgical procedures. Although not yet applicable in the setting of PAL, these measures linking reimbursement to quality of care should refocus physicians' efforts at reducing the incidence of air leak after lung resection.

As noted previously, the monetary costs associated with the presence of a PAL are in part dependent on the treatment strategy selected to address the complication. Much emphasis has been placed on reducing LOS as a means of limiting hospital costs associated with a given procedure. Some investigators feel that adverse surgical outcomes are best defined by risk-adjusted LOS and cost criteria.[17] Physicians may benefit from limiting hospital costs attributed to surgical procedures within their specialty, producing a return on investment for the hospital which, in turn, will look favorably toward funding programmatic growth for the specialty. For thoracic surgical procedures, the use of a predesigned, postoperative care algorithm (fast tracking) decreases LOS and hospital costs.[18–21] These cost-cutting algorithms benefit patients with PAL in a variety of ways. Improved digital monitoring of air leaks,[22,23] the outpatient use of Heimlich valves,[6,19] and use of provocative clamping techniques[24,25] have all led to earlier discharge in this patient population. However, the use of ambulatory chest drainage strategies, such as the Heimlich valve, essentially results in cost shifting from the hospital to the outpatient care setting. From the patient perspective, this strategy may result in direct (visit copayments, medical supply, and transportation costs) and indirect (time off work for loved ones) costs for patients not seen with inpatient treatment. In addition, because patients are not seen daily but rather infrequently with an outpatient strategy, the length of treatment for the PAL (chest tube duration) is likely to be longer than seen in the inpatient setting.

Beyond treatment-associated costs, patients deal with other financial strains related to their illness and exacerbated by the presence of postoperative complications, including PAL. One such strain results from the patients' inability to resume a normal work schedule, particularly if patients are the primary wage earner in the family. Job reassignment, a reduction in wages, or even loss of the job and associated benefits may occur. Ongoing treatment of a postoperative PAL, whether as an inpatient or outpatient, will likely delay the anticipated return-to-work date. The timely ability to return to work for these patients, often with a concomitant diagnosis of cancer, is an underappreciated quality-of-life measure.[26,27]

## IMPACT ON QUALITY AND DELIVERY OF CARE

Even in the best hands, some complications are inevitable following major pulmonary resection,[1,4] a fact accentuated by the overall poor health status of this patient population. Surgeons are acutely aware of *all* morbidity caused by the procedures they perform, and frankly this awareness does not end with the personal questioning and mental anguish caused by our patients' suffering. We are now on the doorstep of generalized public reporting of procedural outcomes, with potential downstream consequences of reduced payment and altered referral patterns. Procedural volume and mortality rates remain hotly debated surrogates of overall quality of care.[28–33] In select thoracic cases, such as LVRS or patients with marginal lung cancer, the development of significant air leaks can lead to mortality or substantial long-term disability. In the Medicare population, it has been suggested that the occurrence of even mild complications, such as air leaks, results in an increase in overall mortality.[34] As with other surgical specialties, overemphasis on certain outcomes measures, such as mortality, can lead thoracic surgeons to change their practice patterns, denying care to individuals who are high risk or need high-risk procedures. One recent study has suggested that although complications occur in low- and high-mortality settings, it is the *response* to the complication rather than the *occurrence* of the complication that determines outcome.[35] This "failure to rescue"[36,37] measure may be a better indicator of quality than the morbidity rate itself.

Even as patients recover from the original complication, such as a prolonged air leak, a lingering influence on the delivery of care remains. The administration of adjuvant chemotherapy is standard of care for patients with resected stage II and III non-small cell lung cancer,[38] and may in the future be recommended for select stage I patients exhibiting poor prognostic markers suggesting a high risk for recurrence.[39] However, despite the reported survival advantages, it is often difficult to initiate and particularly complete the full recommended course of adjuvant therapy because of patient frailty or outright refusal. The pain and slow recovery following lung cancer surgery, particularly via thoracotomy, often makes adjuvant chemotherapy a tough sell to patients. The presence of a prolonged leak (with or without other complications) usually makes the prospect of adjuvant treatment even less appealing. From the physician's perspective, the presence of ongoing thoracostomy drainage for the air leak increases the risk for chemotherapy-related complications, such as empyema or wound infection. These factors, along with the cumulative effects of other comorbidities after resection, may potentially delay or even lead to cancellation of the initiation of adjuvant therapy.

## QUALITY OF LIFE/PATIENT SATISFACTION IMPLICATIONS

Although physicians are primarily focused on the effect of the morbidity and mortality of a surgical procedure, patients are more concerned with long-term functional status after the operation. In a study looking at patient preferences regarding outcome after lung resection, Cykert and colleagues[40] found the possibility of common postoperative complications were unlikely to deter subjects from accepting a thoracic operation. In contrast, subjects perceived significant physical disability extremely undesirable, and this possibility would lead many to reconsider surgical resection. This finding is interesting in that most preoperative predictive models in the literature (mirrored by the preoperative counseling of patients) deal with assessing the risk for acute complications after the surgery. These data would suggest, in the absence of permanent disability resulting from a persistent air leak (quite rare for a parenchymal leak), that the prospect of a PAL would be unlikely to discourage patients from surgical intervention.

Several studies have examined quality of life (QOL) indices in subjects undergoing lung resection. These subjects demonstrate reduced QOL before the surgery compared with the general populace,[41,42] with further decline after the procedure. Opinions vary as to whether QOL returns to preoperative levels[41,43,44] or remains permanently decreased.[42,45] The latter is understandable because most lung surgery is a resectional rather than a restorative procedure.[46] Indeed, some investigators relate the degree of permanent QOL impairment to the extent of lung resection.[45] Given patient preferences,[40] the possibility of a significantly reduced QOL might lead some to reconsider surgical intervention, although others[47] feel concerns over a poor QOL should not deprive patients of the opportunity of curative surgery. Further, reduced QOL before surgery does not predict an increased incidence of postoperative complications.[44,48]

The interplay between complications, quality of life, functional status, and patient satisfaction is complex. Do postoperative complications, such as a prolonged air leak, impact QOL following surgery? Handy and coworkers[42] found that at 6 months there was no correlation between QOL and the degree of postoperative morbidity. Do measures of functional status, which might be adversely affected by postoperative complications, correlate with QOL? It would seem intuitive that QOL would be closely tied to performance on objective tests, such as spirometry or 6-minute walk, although this has not been supported in the literature.[41,42] The only measure possibly predictive of QOL was diffusion capacity for carbon monoxide,[42,44] but this is disputed by others.[41] Finally, what is the cost of postoperative complications to patient satisfaction? Several investigators report a reduced level of patient satisfaction when surgical morbidity is present.[49,50] However, when considering the degree of satisfaction because of the care they received, patients tend to focus on their present state of health, not the relative change of health from before to after an intervention.[51] Thus, the timing of the evaluation is likely important; determining patient satisfaction in the setting of complications just before discharge[49] might lead to spurious findings, compared with satisfaction measured 6 months later.

## SUMMARY

The presence of a prolonged air leak (or any complication) after lung resection generates an array of costs that differ between patients and physicians. These costs can vary depending on the treatment strategy chosen to address the complication. For physicians, concerns about LOS, hospital costs, impact on program growth within a health care system, and quality of care likely predominate. Patients are burdened by additional direct and indirect treatment related costs, concerns regarding resumption of employment and financial stability, and long-term QOL avoiding permanent disability. More research is needed to better assess how these factors interact in patients undergoing thoracic surgery.

## REFERENCES

1. Boffa DJ, Allen MS, Grab JD, et al. Data from the society of thoracic surgeons general thoracic surgery database: the surgical management of primary lung tumors. J Thorac Cardiovasc Surg 2008;135:247.
2. Varela G, Jimenez MF, Novoa N, et al. Estimating hospital costs attributable to prolonged air leak in

pulmonary lobectomy. Eur J Cardiothorac Surg 2005;27:329.

3. Abolhoda A, Liu D, Brooks A, et al. Prolonged air leak following radical upper lobectomy. Chest 1998;113:1507.

4. Allen MS, Darling GE, Pechet TTV, et al. Morbidity and mortality of major pulmonary resections in patients with early-stage lung cancer: initial results of the randomized, prospective ACOSOG Z0030 trial. Ann Thorac Surg 2006;81:1013.

5. Brunelli A, Monteverde M, Borri A, et al. Predictors of prolonged air leak after pulmonary lobectomy. Ann Thorac Surg 2004;77:1205.

6. Cerfolio RJ, Bass CS, Pask AH, et al. Predictors and treatment of persistent air leaks. Ann Thorac Surg 2002;73:1727.

7. Linden PA, Bueno R, Colson YL, et al. Lung resection in patients with preoperative FEV1 < 35% predicted. Chest 2005;127:1984.

8. Cho MH, Malhotra A, Donahue DM, et al. Mechanical ventilation and air leaks after lung biopsy for acute respiratory distress syndrome. Ann Thorac Surg 2006;82:261.

9. DeCamp MM, Blackstone EH, Naunheim KS, et al. Patient and surgical factors influencing air leak after lung volume reduction surgery: lessons learned from the national emphysema treatment trial. Ann Thorac Surg 2006;82:197.

10. Okereke I, Murthy SC, Alster JM, et al. Characterization and importance of air leak after lobectomy. Ann Thorac Surg 2005;79:1167.

11. Belda-Sanchis J, Serra-Mitjans M, Iglesias Sentis M, et al. Surgical sealant for preventing air leaks after pulmonary resections in patients with lung cancer. Cochrane Database Syst Rev 2010;1:CD003051.

12. Bardell T, Petsikas D. What keeps postpulmonary resection patients in hospital? Can Respir J 2003;10:86.

13. Irshad K, Feldman LS, Chu VF, et al. Causes of increased length of hospitalization on a general thoracic surgery service: a prospective observational study. Can J Surg 2002;45:264 [erratum appears in Can J Surg 2003;46(6):466; erratum appears in Can J Surg 2004;47(1):69].

14. Brunelli A, Xiume F, Al Refai M, et al. Air leaks after lobectomy increase the risk of empyema but not of cardiopulmonary complications: a case-matched analysis. Chest 2006;130:1150.

15. Centers for Medicare and Medicaid Services Web site. Available at: http://www.cms.hhs.gov. Accessed March 10, 2010.

16. Pronovost PJ, Goeschel CA, Wachter RM. The wisdom and justice of not paying for "preventable complications". JAMA 2008;299:2197.

17. Fry DE, Pine M, Jones BL, et al. Adverse outcomes in surgery: redefinition of postoperative complications. Am J Surg 2009;197:479.

18. Cerfolio RJ, Pickens A, Bass C, et al. Fast-tracking pulmonary resections. J Thorac Cardiovasc Surg 2001;122:318.

19. McKenna RJ Jr, Mahtabifard A, Pickens A, et al. Fast-tracking after video-assisted thoracoscopic surgery lobectomy, segmentectomy, and pneumonectomy. Ann Thorac Surg 2007;84:1663.

20. Wright CD, Wain JC, Grillo HC, et al. Pulmonary lobectomy patient care pathway: a model to control cost and maintain quality. Ann Thorac Surg 1997;64:299.

21. Zehr KJ, Dawson PB, Yang SC, et al. Standardized clinical care pathways for major thoracic cases reduce hospital costs. Ann Thorac Surg 1998;66:914.

22. Brunelli A, Salati M, Refai M, et al. Evaluation of a new chest tube removal protocol using digital air leak monitoring after lobectomy: a prospective randomised trial. Eur J Cardiothorac Surg 2010;37:56.

23. Cerfolio RJ, Bryant AS. The benefits of continuous and digital air leak assessment after elective pulmonary resection: a prospective study. Ann Thorac Surg 2008;86:396.

24. Cerfolio RJ, Minnich DJ, Bryant AS. The removal of chest tubes despite an air leak or a pneumothorax. Ann Thorac Surg 2009;87:1690.

25. Kirschner PA. "Provocative clamping" and removal of chest tubes despite persistent air leak. Ann Thorac Surg 1992;53:740.

26. Hoang CD, Osborne MC, Maddaus MA. Return to work after thoracic surgery: an overlooked outcome measure in quality-of-life studies. Thorac Surg Clin 2004;14:409.

27. Rasmussen DM, Elverdam B. The meaning of work and working life after cancer: an interview study. Psychooncology 2008;17:1232.

28. Birkmeyer JD, Stukel TA, Siewers AE, et al. Surgeon volume and operative mortality in the United States. N Engl J Med 2003;349:2117.

29. Birkmeyer NJ, Birkmeyer JD. Strategies for improving surgical quality – should payers reward excellence or effort? N Engl J Med 2006;354:864.

30. Khuri SF. Quality, advocacy, healthcare policy, and the surgeon. Ann Thorac Surg 2002;74:641.

31. Kozower BD, Stukenborg GJ, Lau CL, et al. Measuring the quality of surgical outcomes in general thoracic surgery: should surgical volume be used to direct patient referrals? Ann Thorac Surg 2008;86:1405.

32. Luft H, Bunker J, Enthoven A. Should operations be regionalized? The empirical relation between surgical volume and mortality. N Engl J Med 1979;301:1364.

33. Treasure T, Utley M, Bailey A, et al. Assessment of whether in-hospital mortality for lobectomy is a useful standard for the quality of lung cancer surgery: retrospective study. BMJ 2003;327:73.

34. Silber JH, Rosenbaum PR, Trudeau ME, et al. Changes in prognosis after the first postoperative complication. Med Care 2005;43:122.

35. Ghaferi AA, Birkmeyer JD, Dimick JB. Variation in hospital mortality associated with inpatient surgery. N Engl J Med 2009;361:1368.

36. Silber JH, Rosenbaum PR, Schwartz JS, et al. Evaluation of the complication rate as a measure of quality of care in coronary artery bypass graft surgery. JAMA 1995;274:317.

37. Silber JH, Williams SV, Krakauer H, et al. Hospital and patient characteristics associated with death after surgery. A study of adverse occurrence and failure to rescue. Med Care 1992;30:615.

38. Pignon J-P, Tribodet H, Scagliotti GV, et al. Lung adjuvant cisplatin evaluation: a pooled analysis by the LACE Collaborative Group. J Clin Oncol 2008; 26:3552.

39. Potti A, Mukherjee S, Petersen R, et al. A genomic strategy to refine prognosis in early-stage non-small-cell lung cancer. N Engl J Med 2006;355:570.

40. Cykert S, Kissling G, Hansen CJ. Patient preferences regarding possible outcomes of lung resection: what outcomes should preoperative evaluations target? Chest 2000;117:1551.

41. Brunelli A, Socci L, Refai M, et al. Quality of life before and after major lung resection for lung cancer: a prospective follow-up analysis. Ann Thorac Surg 2007;84:410.

42. Handy JR, Asaph JW, Skokan L, et al. What happens to patients undergoing lung cancer surgery? Chest 2002;122:21.

43. Salati M, Brunelli A, Xiume F, et al. Quality of life in the elderly after major lung resection for lung cancer. Interact Cardiovasc Thorac Surg 2009;8:79.

44. Win T, Sharples L, Wells FC, et al. Effect of lung cancer surgery on quality of life. Thorax 2005;60:234.

45. Schulte T, Schniewind B, Dohrmann P, et al. The extent of lung parenchyma resection significantly impacts long-term quality of life in patients with non-small cell lung cancer. Chest 2009;135:322.

46. Mangione CM, Goldman L, Orav EJ, et al. Health-related quality of life after elective surgery: measurement of longitudinal changes. J Gen Intern Med 1997;12:686.

47. McManus K. Concerns of poor quality of life should not deprive patients of the opportunity of curative surgery. Thorax 2003;58:189.

48. Dales RE, Dionne G, Leech JA, et al. Preoperative prediction of pulmonary complications following thoracic surgery. Chest 1993;104:155.

49. Barlesi F, Boyer L, Doddoli C, et al. The place of patient satisfaction in quality assessment of lung cancer thoracic surgery. Chest 2005;128:3475.

50. Bredart A, Coens C, Aaronson N, et al. Determinants of patient satisfaction in oncology settings from European and Asian countries: preliminary results based on the EORTC IN-PATSAT32 questionnaire. Eur J Cancer 2007;43:323.

51. Kane RL, Maciejewski M, Finch M. The relationship of patient satisfaction with care and clinical outcomes. Med Care 1997;35:714.

# Digital and Smart Chest Drainage Systems to Monitor Air Leaks: The Birth of a New Era?

Robert J. Cerfolio, MD[a], Gonzalo Varela, MD, PhD[b],
Alessandro Brunelli, MD[c],*

## KEYWORDS

- Pleural drainage units • Digital chest drainage systems
- Smart suction devices • Pleural air leaks

One of the most elementary aspects of postoperative care after major pulmonary surgery is the proper drainage of the pleural space. The goal is to eliminate all postoperative pleural fluid and air. Prolonged air leak remains one of the most frequent complications after lung resection and all of the surgical staff have to be trained about optimal chest tube management and accurate assessment of air leak size, type, and the presence or absence of postoperative pneumothorax. The measurement or grading of air leaks still relies on a static analog measurement of "bubbles in a chamber." These systems are inherently prone to subjective interpretation and observer variability. Even experienced observers often disagree not only on the size or clinical importance of a leak but sometimes whether one exists or not. These discrepancies occur despite the development, verification, and use of air leak classification systems.[1] Recently, several companies have manufactured and commercialized new pleural drainage units that incorporate electronic components for the digital quantification of air through chest tubes and, in some instances, pleural pressure assessment. The goal of these systems is to objectify this previously subjective bedside clinical parameter and allow for more objective, consistent measurement of air leaks. The belief is this will lead to quicker and more accurate chest tube management. In addition, some systems feature portable suction devices. These may afford earlier mobilization of patients because the pleural drainage chamber is attached to a battery-powered smart suction device. In this article we review clinical experiences using these new devices.

## DIGITAL PLEURAL DRAINAGE SYSTEMS FOR THE MANAGEMENT OF AIR LEAKS

To our knowledge, Thopaz (Medela, Switzerland) and Atmos (Atmosmed, Allentown, PA, USA) are the only 2 commercially available pleural drainage system devices incorporating digital sensors for measuring pleural pressure and flow through the chest tube. Previously manufactured devices are either no longer available (Digivent, Millicore, Sweden) or are experimental systems to be used attached to a conventional drainage set or a Heimlich valve (Airfix, University of Technology, Graz, Sweden).

Both commercially available systems have a built-in screen where instantaneous values of

[a] Section of Thoracic Surgery, Division of Cardiothoracic University, University of Alabama at Birmingham, 703 19th Street, SZRB 736, Birmingham, AL, USA
[b] Service of Thoracic Surgery, Salamanca University Hospital, Paseo San Vicente 58-182, Salamanca, Spain
[c] Division of Thoracic Surgery, Umberto I Regional Hospital, Ospedali Riuniti, Ancona 60020, Italy
* Corresponding author.
*E-mail address:* alexit_2000@yahoo.com

Thorac Surg Clin 20 (2010) 413–420
doi:10.1016/j.thorsurg.2010.03.007
1547-4127/10/$ – see front matter © 2010 Elsevier Inc. All rights reserved.

pleural pressure and flow are shown or their temporal trends can be displayed. Recorded values can also be downloaded to a computer for further analysis.

The clinical usefulness of displaying pressure and flow values has been evaluated in some reports cited later in this article. From a theoretical point of view, these devices can help clinicians to a better understanding of what is going on inside the operated chest because positive pleural pressures can be correlated to persistent pleural air leak or, if no leaks are detected, postoperative pneumothorax can be suspected and treated if necessary. It could be hypothesized that an objective method to detect air leak is superior to a subjective evaluation of the occurrence of bubbling in a chamber and, therefore, decisions on removal of chest tubes are based on scientifically proven evidence. Whether or not these advantages have significant impact in clinical practice is still to be demonstrated.

## PORTABLE SUCTION DEVICES

Most recently, some companies have produced and commercialized chest drainage systems incorporating a stand-alone suction pump allowing these systems to be carried around in the surgical ward. This has the advantage of providing active suction whenever it is needed, giving patients the freedom to ambulate without being attached to wall suction. A point of debate is whether all patients with lung resection would need any suction at all. At the present time the information we have (based on the traditional analog devices) does not permit us to draw any conclusion as to which patients would benefit the most from application of suction, or on which level of active suction should be applied. It is likely that different types of procedures or different characteristics of patients would dictate the need or level of active suction. In this regard, any information derived from digitalized recorded information on air leak flow or pleural pressures will shed more light on this topic. Some studies in the past have shown that passive suction (or gravity mode) is well tolerated by most patients and it is not inferior to active suction in reducing the duration of air leak. Some have advocated the use of alternate regimens with the application of active suction only at night, allowing free mobilization of the patients during the day. This regimen combines the main advantages of both modalities (a moderate level of active suction during the night to favor lung re-expansion, and passive suction during the day to favor mobilization) but it is totally

arbitrary. It is probable that some patients would benefit from more prolonged or more intense active suction regimens and others would benefit from more prolonged periods of passive suction. With the use of portable pumps capable of providing a controlled level of intrapleural pressure, we will have the chance to better study individual patient's responses to externally applied active suction.[2] By using a digitalized system, a recent investigation has shown that, compared with no suction, active suction applied early after pulmonary lobectomy decreased the differential intrapleural pressure after upper lobectomies but had no effect on patients submitted to lower lobectomies. Although the clinical implication of this finding is still to be defined by future investigations, the study has shown the utility to monitor the intrapleural space with digitalized systems capable of providing objective data.

It is worth noting that what we commonly define as no suction or water seal is actually a different form of suction better defined as passive. There is always a certain level of suction or negative pressure differential owing to gravity even when no active suction is applied to the system. The level of this passive suction depends on many factors including the difference in height of the system and the tip of the chest tube inside the chest, but it can be roughly quantified at about 5 to 8 cm $H_2O$. By using portable digital pump devices, this level of pressure can be set and controlled, minimizing variation owing to the position of the device or of the patient and providing more stable conditions that could be beneficial for promoting healing of the lung. More research is needed in this field to better comprehend the role of these devices in clinical daily practice.

## RESULTS OF CLINICAL EXPERIENCE USING DIGITAL DEVICES

The results of all published studies using digital devices are shown in **Table 1** in chronologic order. The AIRFIX (TEUP's Ltd, Deutchlandsberg, Austria) was one of the first digital air leak devices to be used in human patients. Its detailed mechanisms have been previously reported.[3] In summary, the AIRFIX software computes airflow calculations and the data are sent to a hand-held processor that reports a digital reading. A total of 204 patients with an air leak were prospectively enrolled into a clinical trial using AIRFIX by Anegg in 2006.[3] The final report concluded that the device was safe to use and was also more sensitive than the traditionally used device and thus avoided

**Table 1**
Six recent studies evaluating digital chest tube drainage devices, in chronologic order

| Device Used, PI, Year | Type of Study | Number of Pts – Device | Methods | Conclusion |
|---|---|---|---|---|
| AIRFIX Anegg, 2006[3] | Uni-institutional Prospective | 204 pts with air leaks-AIRFIX | Lobe, segment, wedge resection Methods: CT placed on -12 cm | AIRFIX readings consistent, allowed more efficacious removal of CT than traditional system |
| TDS-5L 2007 (unpublished data) | Multi-institutional RCT | 42-TDS-5L 40-Sahara | Lobe, segmentectomy, wedge resection | TDS-5L group- recovered faster, less pain, satisfaction higher for both patient and staff. Observer variability reduced for TDS-5L group. |
| Digivent, Cerfolio, 2008[4] | Uni-institutional RCT | 50-Digivent 50-Sahara | Lobectomy, segment, wedge Methods: CT placed on suction -20 cm on POD 0–1, then placed on water seal | Digivent group had earlier chest tube removal ($P = .034$) and hospital length of stay ($P = .055$) |
| Digivent, Varela, 2009[5] | Uni-institutional RCT | 35-Digivent 26-Analog | Lobectomy, segmentectomy Methods: CT placed to water seal | Concordant readings amongst clinical staff with the digital group was 94% versus 58% in the standard/analog group |
| Digivent, Brunelli, 2009[6] | Uni-Institutional RCT | 82-Digivent 77-Sahara | Lobectomy Methods: CT placed to suction POD 0–1, then alternating suction/water seal | Digivent - Quicker chest tube drainage and discharge |
| Thopaz, Cerfolio, 2009 | Uni-institutional RCT | 48-Thopaz 50-Sahara | Lobectomy, segmentectomy Methods: CT placed on suction -20 cm | Thopaz group: earlier CT removal and earlier hospital discharge |

*Abbreviations:* AL, air leak; CT, chest tube; PI, principal investigator; POD, postoperative day; Pts, patients; RCT, randomized clinical trial.

provocative chest tube clamping before tube removal.

The next 3 series evaluated the Digivent device (Millicore, Sweden). Digivent operates by a single-use electronic sensor with 2 components, one that measures airflow and the other that monitors intrapleural pressure. The readout is presented in a digital display that reports mL/min of air leak. The readout attaches to the top of the canister unit and can be reused for 10 patients. The data can be printed out and stored for documentation and future use. The first published study on the Digivent was published by Cerfolio and Bryant[4] in 2008. Digivent was compared with the standard analog (Sahara Pleurevac, Teleflex, Research Triangle Park, NC, USA) chest tube drainage system. This was a prospective randomized clinical trial on 100 patients. Inclusion criteria mandated that all patients who underwent pulmonary resection were randomized to either the digital device or the analog group. One unique aspect of this study design was a 1-hour crossover, where patients with an air leak were placed on both devices and the readings evaluated for correlation. Consequently, a linear correlation was found between the RDC analog air leak scale when compared with the digital scale (**Fig. 1**). This was the first study to show the correlation between digital air leaks and a clinically validated classification system for air leaks. Other findings of that study were that patients randomized to the digital system experienced significantly reduced chest tube duration ($P = .030$), and there was less observer discordance and a marginally reduced hospital length of stay ($P = .055$).

Varela and colleagues[5] in 2009 reported the findings of a randomized control study evaluating the use of the Digivent to a traditional water seal chamber device in 54 post-thoracotomy patients. All patients underwent pulmonary lobectomy, segmentectomy, or wedge resection and were placed on water seal following surgery. Varela and his team[5] observed a concordance rate between observers for air leak rating of only 58% in the traditional water seal chamber device group compared with a 94% concordance rate in the Digivent group. These findings led to improved chest tube management in patients randomized to the digital device.

Brunelli and colleagues[6] in 2009 were the third group to report their findings using the Digivent. They performed a uni-institutional randomized study to assess the effectiveness of a new fast-track chest tube removal protocol taking advantage of digital monitoring of air leak compared with the same analog device used by us (the Saharah Pleuravac, Teleflex). In this series, 166 patients who underwent lobectomy were randomized to 2 groups. The first group had their chest tube removed based on digitally recorded measurements of air leak flow. The second group had their chest tubes removed based on instantaneous assessment of air leakage on daily rounds using the traditional analog system. Brunelli and colleagues[6] showed the patients in the digital group had greater mean reductions in chest tube duration ($P<.001$), hospital stay ($P = .007$) of 0.9 day, and a greater average cost savings per patient ($P = .008$). Additionally, 51% of patients with the digital drainage device had their chest tube removed by the second postoperative day compared with only 12% of those with the analog device.

The fifth study on digital air leaks is a pilot multi-institutional randomized clinical trial that featured the TDS-5L (Medela, Switzerland) in 2007. This system was the first prototype from Medela and the predecessor of the Thopaz. The primary goal of this study was to compare the efficacy, safety, and clinician satisfaction of the TDS-5L digital system that featured both a bubble chamber and digital measurement of air leaks. Outcomes of patients on the digital TDS-5L system were compared with those of patients who received the standard Sahara analog system. The study showed that patients who had a Medela TD5-SL tended toward earlier chest tube removal and treatment period compared with patients with the

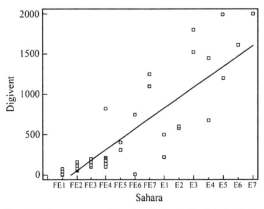

**Fig. 1.** Linear regression for Robert David Cerfolio (RDC; Sahara S-11,000, Teleflex, Research Triangle Park, NC) system versus the digital (Digivent, Millicore, Sweden) system ($r2 = 0.80$; regression equation: $y = 2.094 + 0.0061x$). E, expiratory; FE, forced expiratory. (*Reprinted from* Cerfolio RJ, Bryant AS. The benefit of continuous and digital air leak assessment after elective pulmonary resection: a prospective study. Ann Thorac Surg 2008;86:362–7; with permission from The Society of Thoracic Surgeons.)

analog device. Another finding was that patients who were randomized to the digital group were significantly more mobile as compared with those patients in the traditional group.

The sixth and final study on digital devices comes from University of Alabama.[7] Cerfolio and colleagues evaluated the newest digital chest tube drainage device, the Thopaz, in 2008 in a prospective clinical trial. All 98 patients underwent posterior lateral thoracotomy with pulmonary resection and were randomized to have their chest tubes placed to the Sahara Pleuravac (Teleflex), which features a 7-column air-leak meter or to the Thopaz. Typically one chest tube was placed for lobectomy and chest tubes were placed to −20 cm suction per study protocol on the day of surgery and then placed to water seal. If an air leak was detected on morning rounds the size and type of the leak was recorded based on either the RDC or the Thopaz digital system by 2 different clinicians at the same time. Chest tubes were removed when the output was less than 450 mL/d and air leak was 20 mL/min or less on the digital system or nondiscernable on the analog system. Clinician satisfaction with the 2 different devices was assessed by asking the nurse, patient, and physician a series of questions that included the following: ease of ambulation with the device, the quietness of the unit, the set-up time, the degree of variability of scoring air leaks, and overall satisfaction. Patients randomized to the Thopaz device had slightly reduced duration of chest tubes (3.0 days for digital device compared with 4.5 days for the analog group, $P = .042$) and length of stay (3.9 days for digital group and 4.6 days for analog group, $P = .153$). Three patients on the Thopaz unit were discharged home on postoperative day 4 (POD 4) with their chest tubes in place. Five patients in the analog group went home on an Atrium Express (Hudson, NH, USA) on POD 4 or 5. Patients who went home on the digital device were able to convey their air leak status to our clinical team over the phone more easily than those on the analog system and one patient returned 2 weeks sooner than the planned date for chest tube removable. Additionally, patients found it significantly easier to ambulate with the digital device as compared with the analog device ($P<.001$). The patient and clinician satisfaction between the 2 different types of drainage and air leak systems was not significantly different. One common complaint with the Thopaz system was the inability to troubleshoot alarms, but this complaint decreased as the staff became more experienced with the digital unit. In addition, there was greater observer agreement about air leaks ($P = .002$).

## COMMENT

We live in a world that has become increasingly digitalized and we have become reliant on technological equipment in all facets of our lives. As physicians, we and our patients are surrounded with advanced machinery, most of which improves the care we deliver to our patients. However, it also increases the cost. The days of holding a glass thermometer to the light to interpret where the line of mercury is best located to determine a patient's temperature has been replaced by the more accurate, reproducible and easier to read digital thermometer. Digital air leak devices have done the same for the measurement of air leaks out of chest tubes. Before these systems, even the presence or absence of an air leak at times was difficult to ascertain using even the best analog systems. Is it not infrequently that one observer reports an air leak because of a perceived bubble or swing in a chamber in a drainage system whereas another physician present during the exact same examination reported no air leak.

Air leaks remain a vexing and important clinical problem. They are not just an annoyance that delays discharge but in addition they are a surrogate marker and even perhaps the cause of increased morbidity for some complications such as pneumonia, subcutaneous emphysema, atrial fibrillation, and increased hospital stay.[8] Any technology that improves our ability to treat alveolar pleural fistulas (air leaks) in a scientific, objective manner is an important clinical accomplishment and will most likely translate into better care for patients and into cost savings for hospitals.

This review of the current literature has shown that digital devices improve chest tube management and patient care. The ideal characteristics of a chest tube drainage system after pulmonary resection have been elucidated in the past[4] but include the following: has a large environmental friendly reservoir for fluid collection and analysis; is able to exert different levels of suction; is compact to permit patient ambulation; is latex free, quiet, tip-over safe, reusable, and inexpensive; can digitally and continuously and accurately measure the amount of chest tube drainage and the size of air leaks; produces a written record of events in the pleural space; is easy for both staff and patients to use; allows for the patient to be sent home on the same device owing to persistent leak; and allows data to be relayed to the nurses' station or physician's office for assessment. No current system delivers all of these characteristics.

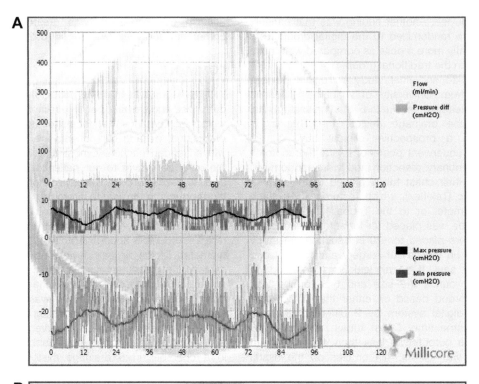

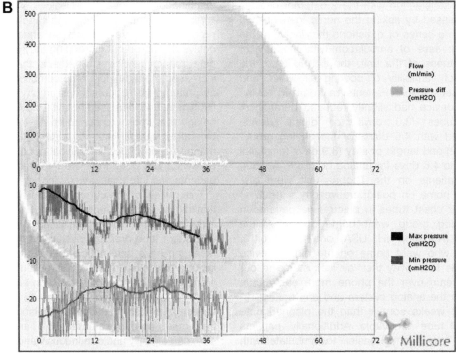

**Fig. 2.** Pleural pressures and flow through chest tube after lobectomy. In case A, after 36 hours of hospitalization, the patient could be discharged home because a decreasing trend cannot be observed. Case B shows decreasing values of air leak and pleural pressures. Early chest tube withdrawal can be expected after the first 24 hours.

The decision that each physician and hospital administrator must decide is which system is most cost effective and for which patient a digital drainage system improves patient care and still reduces cost. For example, is it best to apply a digital system to all patients immediately postoperatively? Or, should they be reserved only for those with risk factors for prolonged air leaks or those with air leaks on POD 1 or 2 who are failing standard treatment algorithms of chest tubes using an analog system? These are the key questions that will determine the eventual distribution and clinical use of digital chest drainage devices. We, as well as others, have shown that most patients with air leaks can be managed, fast-tracked, and enjoy safe results with a 3- or 4-day postoperative stay using the analog system[9]; however, the digital system offers unique advantages.

Many of the studies listed in this review had similar findings. These include greater concordance rates about the presence and size of air leaks, shorter chest tube duration, shorter hospital stay, and more consistent, objective (and even more sensitive) readings of air leaks as compared with the analog "bubble" devices. For example, the Thopaz detected air leaks as low as 20 mL/min, which were found to be clinically insignificant and chest tubes were removed safely with air leaks this size. We have not been able to duplicate findings using any analog air leak system over the past several years. Some studies have shown digital systems are cost effective as well by reducing the hospital length of stay and chest tube duration. The Digivent, TDS-5L, and Thopaz systems allow for the ability to plot the size of air leaks and intrapleural pressure over time so that the trend of the size of the air leak can been determined. A final important conclusion of this review is that in using the digital chest tube systems, the assessment of air leaks can become something the nurse or even patients themselves can read to a physician over the phone. Reporting air leaks no longer requires an experienced physician at the bedside and thus more rapid chest tube management decisions can be made.

There are theoretical advantages of measuring pressures in the pleural space. For example, **Fig. 2** depicts 2 printouts obtained with the no longer available Digivent system. Both correspond to patients after lobectomy for lung cancer. In the upper part of the figure, a trend toward a persistent air leak is observed, whereas in the other case, a rapid decrease of pressures and flow are evident after 24 hours. In the first case, the patient could be discharged home sooner with a chest tube after a postoperative in-hospital period of 36 to 72 hours because it is unlikely the tube could be removed safely if the leak is not healing.

There is little doubt in our opinion that our future is the digital and continuous assessment of air leaks and of the pleural space. Digital drainage devices provide another accurate assessment of an important patient sign at the bedside. A digital system allows the nursing and resident staff, regardless of their level of education or training to be able to report a patient's air leak status over the phone or in the chart. The ability of the digital chest tube drainage device to provide a medical record will also help protect the physician and nurse medical-legally. In the future it is very conceivable that on rounds the physician will simply place his or her cellular phone near the device and download the air leak curves to it. In patients who are sent home on a digital device the information may be able to be transmitted over the phone lines as is currently done with pacemakers. We are already able to download air leak data to a laptop computer at the nurses' station and display the current size of the air leak and its trend based on the chest tube settings. The assimilation rate of this technology will ultimately come down to the cost of the device, the number of patients who benefit from it by having earlier discharge, and the advantage of quicker chest tube removal. This will depend heavily on each surgeon's bias toward chest tube management, their typical length of stay, and other habits that they may or may not be willing to challenge and change.

In conclusion, this review of the current literature concerning digital air leak pleural drainage systems has shown that the devices are safe. They provide consistent and reliable detection of air leaks and report air leaks in mL/min and this scale correlates with the only validated classification system for air leaks previously reported on analog systems. It objectifies some of the subjective aspects of air leak detection and sizing and thus improves chest tube management. This shortens hospital stay by leading to earlier chest tube removal in patients with air leaks. However, the cost savings are not yet fully defined. Carefully designed studies that examine actual cost, charges, and saving of these devices given their more expensive initial price tag are needed and are already under way.

## REFERENCES

1. Cerfolio RJ. Advances in thoracostomy tube management. Surg Clin North Am 2002;82:833–48.
2. Varela G, Brunelli A, Jimenez MF, et al, Chest drainage suction decreases differential pleural pressure after

upper lobectomy and has no effect after lower lobectomy. Eur J Cardiothorac Surg 2010;37:531–4.

3. Anegg U, Lindenmann J, Matzi V, et al. AIRFIX: the first digital postoperative chest tube airflowmetry—a novel method to quantify air leakage after lung resection. Eur J Cardiothorac Surg 2006;29: 867–72.

4. Cerfolio RJ, Bryant AS. The benefit of continuous and digital air leak assessment after elective pulmonary resection: a prospective study. Ann Thorac Surg 2008;86:362–7.

5. Varela G, Jimenez MF, Novoa NM, et al. Postoperative chest tube management: measuring air leak using an electronic device decreases variability in the clinical practice. Eur J Cardiothorac Surg 2009;35:28–31.

6. Brunelli A, Salati M, Refai M, et al. Evaluation of a new chest tube removal protocol using direct air leak monitoring after lobectomy: a prospective randomized trial. Eur J Cardiothorac Surg 2010;37:56–60.

7. Cerfolio RJ, Bryant AS. The quantification of postoperative air leak. DOI:10.1510/mmcts.2007.003129.

8. Cerfolio RJ, Bass CS, Pask AH, et al. Predictors and treatment of persistent air leaks. Ann Thorac Surg 2002;73:1727–31.

9. Cerfolio RJ, Pickens A, Bass CS, et al. Fast-tracking pulmonary resection. J Thorac Cardiovasc Surg 2001;122:318–24.

# Portable Chest Drainage Systems and Outpatient Chest Tube Management

Gonzalo Varela, MD, PhD, FETCS*,
Marcelo F. Jiménez, MD, PhD, FETCS, Nuria Novoa, MD, PhD

**KEYWORDS**

- Ambulatory pleural drainage management
- Postoperative air leak • Heimlich valve

The management of outpatient pleural problems has been reported in the literature in diseases such as uncomplicated spontaneous pneumothorax[1] and chronic malignant or infectious pleural effusions, with favorable results.[2,3] Outpatient management of prolonged air leak after lung volume reduction has also been reported.[4]

This article addresses the topic of outpatient pleural drainage management after major thoracic procedures, focusing on outpatient management of prolonged air leak after pulmonary lobectomy. This topic has been also studied previously but it encompasses some controversial aspects.

The aims of this article are to review previously published experiences, indications, reported adverse events, and available tools for outpatient pleural drainage and fluid collection.

## RATIONALE FOR DISCHARGING PATIENTS UNDERGOING PLEURAL DRAINAGE

Concerns about cost containment have forced surgeons to introduce some changes in their practice to reduce expenses while trying not to compromise on the quality of patient care. Shortening hospital stay (HS) after lung resection has been reported as an effective measure to reduce the costs of this surgical procedure,[5,6] and its practice is not associated with an increase in emergency readmissions.[7] However, shortening HS has been criticized by some authors who consider that for most patients, the costs directly attributable to the last day of a hospital stay are an economically insignificant component of the total costs[8] and that shortening HS simply shifts costs to outpatient care facilities.[9]

Some experiences in fast-tracking pulmonary resection using the conventional[10] or video-assisted approach[11] have shown that HS can be considerably reduced, keeping outcomes and patient satisfaction at a high level of quality. One of the measures included in fast-tracking protocols is home discharge with pleural drainage in cases with prolonged air leak (PAL). Because PAL is one of the most prevalent complications after lung resection,[12] discharging these patients undergoing chest drainage is expected to have a positive influence on saving many nonuseful hospital days[13] and decrease hospital costs.

This idea has to be approached with caution because postoperative chest drainage management is usually based not on scientific data but on the team preference toward conventional protocols and time-honored practice;[14] therefore, any changes affecting nursing perioperative protocols cannot be implemented without some investment in training the ward and outpatient clinic staff to ensure convenient care for patients.

## DISCHARGE CRITERIA AND CHEST TUBE MANAGEMENT

A few reports describing criteria for discharging patients undergoing chest drainage and outcomes

Service of Thoracic Surgery, Salamanca University Hospital, Paseo San Vicente, 58-182 Salamanca, Spain
* Corresponding author.
E-mail address: gvs@usal.es

Thorac Surg Clin 20 (2010) 421–426
doi:10.1016/j.thorsurg.2010.03.006

of ambulatory PAL management after major lung resection have been published (**Table 1**).[11,13,15–17]

Discharge criteria are described in the papers by Rieger and colleagues[13] and Cerfolio and colleagues[17] These investigators underline that willingness of the patient to be discharged home wearing a chest tube and the patient's understanding of the functioning of the system are mandatory. According to the article by Rieger and colleagues[13] the patient has to fulfill several additional criteria to be discharged home: appropriate distance to medical support, reasonable control of pain, and no marginal pulmonary function. Marginal pulmonary function is an exclusion criteria for Cerfolio and colleagues,[17] and it is defined as forced expiratory volume of air in 1 second ($FEV_1\%$) of less than 50 or lung diffusion capacity for carbon monoxide (DLCO%) of less than 80. These investigators recommend testing the patient's compliance with the device and the absence of major pneumothorax and/or subcutaneous emphysema clinically and at a chest radiograph taken after 6 hours with the device connected to the chest tube and without suction. An apical pneumothorax is not considered a contraindication for ambulatory management.

In all published case series, patients are scheduled for outpatient consultation after discharge and are recommended to call the surgeon's office if they experience any problems related to the procedure.

No major complications have been reported in the literature directly related to the outpatient management of chest tubes after lung resection. The rate of emergency readmissions ranged from 2.2% to 8.3%, and most readmissions (6 out of 9 reported cases) were due to pleural empyema with or without pneumonia. In a retrospective matched analysis,[18] PAL over 7 days has been correlated to a higher rate of pleural empyema compared with patients without air leak or those having air leakage for less than 7 days. Although there are no scientifically proven data on the effectiveness of antibiotic prophylaxis to prevent pleural empyema related to PAL, some investigators[17] recommend treating patients with antibiotics up to the time of tube withdrawal.

Suction is not necessary for ambulatory patients with PAL. The usefulness of suction after pulmonary lobectomy has been debated in the literature, and a systematic review[19] concluded that there is no evidence of the advantages of postoperative suction except in cases with massive air leak,

**Table 1**
**Reported experiences in the outpatient management of prolonged air leak after pulmonary resection**

| References | Number of Cases | Device Used | Readmission Rate and Causes | Duration of Outpatient Chest Tube Management in Days, Range (Mean) |
|---|---|---|---|---|
| Rieger et al[13] | 36 | 500 mL dry chest drainage unit | 3 (8.3%) Pneumothorax, localized empyema, pain control | 3–36 (11.2) |
| Ponn et al[15] | 45 | Heimlich valve | 1 (2.2%) Pneumonia and parapneumonic effusion | 3–23 (7.8) |
| Lodi and Stefani[16] | 18 | Original device using one-way valve and plastic bag | 0 | 4–32 (11.5) |
| Cerfolio et al[17] | 194 | Heimlich valve or 500 mL dry chest drainage unit | 22 (11.3%) Scheduled overnight readmission for provocative clamping and withdraw: 14 (7.2%) Emergency readmissions: 5 (2.6%) 3 pleural empyema 1 pain control 1 pneumonia | Data not provided |

and that this is a contraindication for home discharge.

In our practice, a visit to the outpatient clinic is scheduled 1 week after hospital discharge (**Fig. 1**). At that time, the presence of air leak is checked and the tube withdrawn if there is no bubbling during expiratory maneuvers. Besides checking for the presence of bubbling through the tube, the patient is interviewed and a physical examination performed to rule out the obstruction

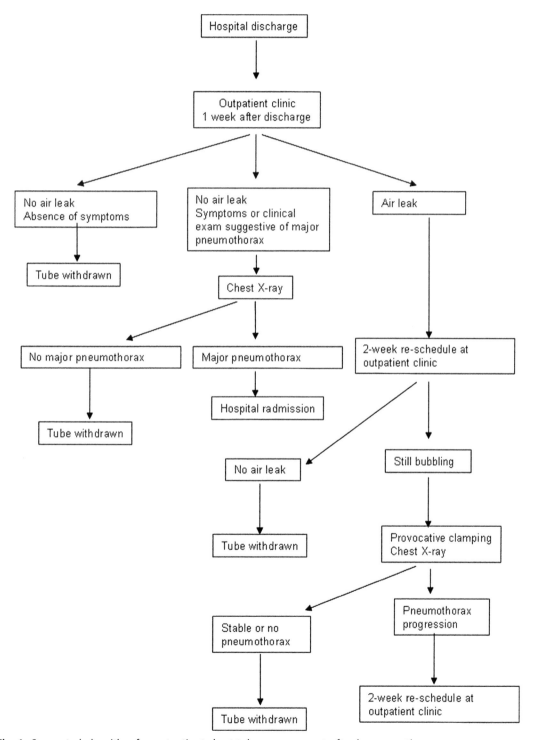

**Fig. 1.** Suggested algorithm for outpatient chest tube management after lung resection.

**Table 2**
Commercially available devices for outpatient plural drainage after lung resection

| Type of Device | Advantages | Disadvantages | Manufacturers[a] |
|---|---|---|---|
| One-way valve without reservoir (Heimlich valves) | Inexpensive and simple | Pleural fluid spillage<br>Patient-induced malposition is possible[b]<br>Valve malfunctioning in presence of blood clots | Vygon (France)<br>BD Bard-Parker (LSA)<br>Infusion Concepts (USA) |
| One-way valve with small reservoir | Simple<br>Avoid pleural fluid spillage<br>Air leak check device<br>Malposition is not possible | More expensive than Heimlich valves | Atrium Medical Corp (USA) |
| One-way valve with 1500 mL soft reservoir | Inexpensive | Suction is not possible if needed during follow-up | Smiths Medical (UK)[c] |
| One-way valve with 500 mL hard case reservoir | Air leak check device<br>Suction is possible if needed<br>High output of air and fluid can be drained if needed | Expensive | Atrium Medical Co'rp (USA)<br>Teleflex Medical Inc (USA) |

[a] This is not an exhaustive list.
[b] Except in the model manufactured by Infusion Concepts, which incorporates a Luer lock system for chest tube and valve connection.
[c] Not available in the United States.

of the tube and the occurrence of a major pneumothorax. If this situation is suspected, a chest radiograph is taken and the patient readmitted if a major pneumothorax is found.

In the case of persistent air leakage, the patient is rescheduled for a further visit after 2 weeks, and the status of the pleural leakage is checked again. In the presence of a small flow during expiratory maneuvers, the tube is clamped and a chest radiograph is taken 2 hours later. If there is no pneumothorax or in the absence of progression of a previous pneumothorax chamber, the tube is withdrawn.

The presence of an air leak is usually considered a contraindication for removal of a chest tube. In a recently published article by Cerfolio and colleagues,[17] the safety of chest tube removal in patients with persistent air leak was investigated. The investigators concluded that chest tubes can be safely removed even if the patients have a pneumothorax, if the following criteria are met: the patients have been asymptomatic, they have no subcutaneous emphysema after 14 days on a portable device at home, and the pleural space deficit has not increased in size. Several published articles confirm the idea that residual pleural spaces after lung resection are not a major threat to the health of the patient and in many cases, can be left untreated to avoid iatrogenic complications.[20,21]

We were unable to find any recommendations in the literature on the maximum distance between the patient's home and the hospital that can be considered safe for patients discharged with pleural drainage. In our experience, almost half of the patients who were discharged with portable chest drainage systems lived more than 100 km from the center, and in 25% of the cases, the distance was more than 200 km. Distance-related problems did not arise. In our series, the rate of emergency readmissions was 7% (3 cases), and 2 of the patients had to be readmitted because of pneumonia and pleural empyema (1 case each). It is our policy that all patients being discharged with portable pleural drainage devices are given written information on the fundamental points to be borne in mind. As an additional measure of security, nursing staff in the medical facilities closest to the patient's home are also informed about the particulars of the patient.

## AVAILABLE DEVICES FOR OUTPATIENT PLEURAL DRAINAGE MANAGEMENT

The types and some of the commercially available devices for ambulatory pleural drainage are summarized in **Table 2**. Indwelling pleural catheters for chronic evacuation of malignant pleural effusions have not been considered because this is beyond the scope of this article.

The Heimlich valve is the simplest method of outpatient pleural drainage. Some problems related to patient-induced malposition of the valve, leading to tension pneumothorax and emergency readmission, have been published in the literature.[22,23] Fortunately, these problems are rare, and the reliability of flutter valves for pleural drainage after lung resection has been demonstrated in the literature.[24-27] The main inconvenience of the Heimlich valve is pleural fluid spillage, which is bothersome for the patient and his environment. To avoid this problem, the valve should be attached to a perforated plastic bag, or a specifically designed one-way valve including a small reservoir can be used.[28] Outside the United States, a device including a flutter valve and a plastic bag with a vent is available.[26]

Some small, conventional, chest drainage units useful for outpatient management are also available.[13] These units have the advantage of incorporating a system for checking air leaks and the possibility of suction if this is needed in the follow-up period. However, they are more expensive than a classic Heimlich valve or a plastic bag.

## SUMMARY

Ambulatory chest drainage after lung resection is a safe procedure if patients are selected according to previously established criteria. The rate of expected emergency readmissions is low, and no major problems have been reported. There are several devices available on the market facilitating ambulatory pleural space management, and the adoption of this procedure depends on local criteria.

## REFERENCES

1. Hassani B, Foote J, Borgundvaag B. Outpatient management of primary spontaneous pneumothorax in the emergency department of a community hospital using a small-bore catheter and a Heimlich valve. Acad Emerg Med 2009;16:513–8.
2. Tremblay A, Michaud G. Single-centre experience with 250 tunnelled pleural catheter insertions for malignant pleural effusion. Chest 2006;129:362–8.
3. Davies HE, Rahman NM, Parker RJ, et al. Use of indwelling pleural catheters for chronic pleural infection. Chest 2008;133:546–9.
4. McKenna RJ Jr, Fischel RJ, Brenner M, et al. Use of the Heimlich valve to shorten hospital stay after lung reduction surgery for emphysema. Ann Thorac Surg 1996;61:1115–7.

5. Wright CD, Wain JC, Grillo HC, et al. Pulmonary lobectomy patient care pathway: a model to control cost and maintain quality. Ann Thorac Surg 1997;64: 299–302.

6. Zehr KJ, Yang SC, Heitmillor RF. Standadized clinical care pathways for major thoracic cases reduce hospital costs. Ann Thorac Surg 1998;66:914–9.

7. Varela G, Aranda LJ, Jiménez MF, et al. Emergency hospital readmission after major lung resection: prevalence and related variables. Eur J Cardiothorac Surg 2004;26:494–7.

8. Taheri PA, Butz DA, Greenfield LJ. Length of stay has minimal impact on the cost of hospital admission. J Am Coll Surg 2000;191:123–30.

9. Weingarten S, Riedinger MS, Sndhu M, et al. Can practice guidelines safely reduce hospital length of stay? Results from a multicenter interventional study. Am J Med 1998;105:33–40.

10. Cerfolio RJ, Pickens A, Bass C, et al. Fast-tracking pulmonary resections. J Thorac Cardiovasc Surg 2001;122:318–24.

11. McKenna RJ Jr, Mahtabifard A, Pickens A, et al. Fast-tracking after video-assisted thoracoscopic surgery lobectomy, segmentectomy, and pneumonectomy. Ann Thorac Surg 2007;84:1663–7.

12. Okereke I, Murthy SC, Alster JM, et al. Characterization and importance of air leak after lobectomy. Ann Thorac Surg 2005;79:1167–73.

13. Rieger KM, Wroblewski HA, Brooks JA, et al. Postoperative outpatient chest tube management: initial experience with a new portable system. Ann Thorac Surg 2007;84:630–2.

14. Mattioli S, Berrisford RG, Lugaresi ML, et al. Survey on chest drainage systems adopted in Europe. Interact Cardiovasc Thorac Surg 2008;7: 1155–9.

15. Ponn RB, Silverman HJ, Federico JA. Outpatient chest tube management. Ann Thorac Surg 1997; 64:1437–40.

16. Lodi R, Stefani A. A new portable chest drainage device. Ann Thorac Surg 2000;69:998–1001.

17. Cerfolio RJ, Minnich DJ, Bryant AS. The removal of chest tubes despite an air leak or a pneumothorax. Ann Thorac Surg 2009;87:1690–6.

18. Brunelli A, Xiume F, Al Refai M, et al. Air leaks after lobectomy increase the risk of empyema but not of cardiopulmonary complications: a case-matched analysis. Chest 2006;130:1150–6.

19. Sanni A, Critchley A, Dunning J. Should chest drains be put on suction or not following pulmonary lobectomy? Interact Cardiovasc Thorac Surg 2006; 5:275–8.

20. Misthos P, Kokotsakis J, Konstantinou M, et al. Postoperative residual pleural spaces: characteristics and natural history. Asian Cardiovasc Thorac Ann 2007;15:54–8.

21. Barker WL. Natural history of residual air spaces after pulmonary resection. Chest Surg Clin N Am 1996;6:585–613.

22. Crocker HL, Ruffin RE. Patient-induced complications of a Heimlich flutter valve. Chest 1998;113: 838–9.

23. Mariani PJ, Sharma S. Iatrogenic tension pneumothorax complicating outpatient Heimlich valve chest drainage. J Emerg Med 1994;12:477–9.

24. Waller DA, Edwards JG, Rajesh PB. A physiological comparison of flutter valve drainage bags and underwater seal systems for postoperative air leaks. Thorax 1999;54:442–3.

25. Rathinam S, Steyn RS. Management of complicated postoperative air-leak - a new indication for the Asherman chest seal. Interact Cardiovasc Thorac Surg 2007;6:691–4.

26. McManus KG, Spence GM, McGuigan JA. Outpatient chest tubes. Ann Thorac Surg 1998;66:299–300.

27. Graham ANJ, Cosgrove AP, Gibbons JRP, et al. Randomised clinical trial of chest drainage systems. Thorax 1992;47:461–2.

28. Abdul Rahman MR, Min Joanna OS, Fikri AM, et al. Pocket-sized Heimlich valve (Pneumostat) after bullae resection: a 5-year review. Ann Thorac Surg 2009;88:979–81.

# Special Situations: Air Leak After Lung Volume Reduction Surgery and in Ventilated Patients

Saila P. Nicotera, MD, MPH[a], Malcolm M. Decamp, MD[b],*

## KEYWORDS

- Prolonged air leak • Lung volume reduction surgery
- Severe emphysema • Barotrauma • Volutrauma
- Mechanical ventilation

Patients undergoing lung volume reduction surgery (LVRS) and those supported by mechanical ventilation are among our most vulnerable patients. Prolonged air leak in these fragile patients can have dire and fatal consequences. This article describes the incidence of prolonged air leak in these populations, the causes ascribed to their development, and strategies that may be applied to their prevention and treatment.

## PROLONGED AIR LEAK AFTER LVRS

LVRS originated in the work of Brantigan and colleagues,[1] published in 1959. The operation received little attention but was resurrected by Cooper and colleagues[2] in 1993. It became a meaningful treatment of severe emphysema during the 1990s. The theoretical benefits included reduction in airway resistance by restoring lung elastic recoil and the tethering function on small airways; restoration of normal chest wall recoil; improved ventilation-perfusion matching; and reduction in end-expiratory volume, allowing for optimized diaphragmatic excursion and generation of negative intrathoracic pressure.[3,4] LVRS

has been shown to be beneficial in even the most severely afflicted patients.[2,3]

Additions and adjustments were made to the original techniques but, despite the revisions, prolonged air leak remains the most common complication after LVRS. The consequences of leak are significant, resulting in longer hospital stay, readmission to the intensive care unit, prolonged need for tube thoracostomy and adjunctive treatments, and even a higher rate of infectious and cardiopulmonary complications.[5] This article describe the incidence of prolonged air leak after LVRS, examines the risk factors and mechanisms at play, and reviews the various techniques that have been used to reduce its occurrence.

## INCIDENCE OF PROLONGED AIR LEAK AFTER LVRS

Prolonged air leak is generally defined as a leak lasting 7 days or more. It is estimated that prolonged air leaks after LVRS occur in 46% to 80% of cases.[2,6] In the National Emphysema Treatment Trial (NETT), in which 552 patients underwent bilateral, stapled LVRS, the incidence of prolonged air leak was 50%.[5] An examination of operative

The authors have nothing to disclose.
[a] Department of Surgery, Beth Israel Deaconess Medical Center, 110 Francis Street, Suite 9B, Boston, MA 02215, USA
[b] Division of Thoracic Surgery, Northwestern Memorial Hospital, Northwestern University Feinberg School of Medicine, 676 North Saint Clair Street, Suite 650, Chicago, IL 60611, USA
* Corresponding author.
E-mail address: mdecamp@nmh.org

Thorac Surg Clin 20 (2010) 427–434
doi:10.1016/j.thorsurg.2010.04.003
1547-4127/10/$ – see front matter © 2010 Elsevier Inc. All rights reserved.

approach reveals that the prolonged air leak rate does not differ among patients undergoing median sternotomy, thoracotomy, or thoracoscopy for lung volume reduction.[6–8] This finding was borne out in the analysis of prolonged air leak undertaken in the NETT trial.[5]

## EARLY ATTEMPTS TO REDUCE LEAK

Several attempts at reducing the incidence of prolonged air leak were made. In one of the earliest articles on the subject, Cooper[9] noted that air leaks occurred most often at the proximal staple line intraoperatively, and that using a stapling device buttressed with strips of bovine pericardium was found to eliminate these leaks, as shown by intraoperative underwater testing. A randomized trial comparing buttressed with nonbuttressed staple lines showed that the buttressed group had significantly fewer air leaks overall, but there were no significant differences in the incidence of prolonged air leak or in the rates of reoperation for prolonged air leak.[10,11] In an outcomes study comparing a nonresectional LVRS technique with traditional resectional techniques, neither the resected nor the unresected group used buttressing or other reinforcement techniques, but the leak rates were as low or lower than the rates reported in buttressed groups.[12] In addition, buttressing staple lines with bovine pericardium has resulted in complications of interstitial pneumonia, pseudotumor formation, recurrent hemoptysis, staple/strip-optysis, and obstructive pneumonia.[13] These are presumably due to a significant inflammatory reaction stimulated by the material.

Similarly, a randomized comparison of laser bullectomy with stapled LVRS for diffuse emphysema revealed no significant differences in rates of prolonged air leak, although significantly more patients in the laser group developed late pneumothorax.[14]

Pleural tents created intraoperatively were shown to reduce the incidence of prolonged air leak in a small study of 8 emphysematous patients, 2 of whom underwent LVRS. The other 8 underwent bullectomy. Parietal pleura overlying the resected portions of lung were used as staple-line reinforcement. No prolonged air leak was seen in this study.[15] However, examination of the 60 patients in the NETT trial who underwent pleural tent creation showed no significant difference in the rate of prolonged air leak.[5] Sealants and glues for preventing prolonged air leak in pulmonary resections have been studied with varying results.[16] However, data from the NETT trial focusing exclusively on LVRS patients show no clear benefit of adjunctive procedures to reduce the incidence of prolonged air leak.

In short, buttressing pleural tent creation, sealants, glues, pleurodesis, laser bullectomy have been shown to reduce the incidence of prolonged air leak after LVRS.

## WHY PROLONGED AIR LEAKS OCCUR AFTER LVRS

In a study of prolonged air leak after pulmonary resection by Brunelli and colleagues,[17] a large series of patients undergoing lobectomy or bilobectomy for non–small-cell lung cancer were analyzed. Patients at greatest risk for developing prolonged air leak were those with a lower mean forced expiratory volume in 1 second ($FEV_1$; 79% vs 90%), lower mean forced vital capacity (FVC), lower $FEV_1$/FVC ratio (0.66 vs 0.71), lower predicted postoperative $FEV_1$ (63% vs 72%), those with adhesions (51% vs 30%), and those undergoing upper lobe resections (74% vs 63%). In short, emphysematous lung parenchyma rendered patients undergoing pulmonary resection for cancer vulnerable to developing prolonged air leaks. Patients undergoing LVRS (a set of patients with severe emphysema) have the highest rates of prolonged air leak of any group undergoing pulmonary resection. The findings of Brunelli and colleagues[17] were closely mirrored in the NETT trial identification of independent risk factors for developing prolonged air leak. These included upper lobe resection, the presence of tenacious adhesions, and low carbon monoxide diffusion in the lung (DLCO). Inhaled steroid use was also found to be an independent predictor of leak duration, ostensibly due to trapping of steroids in the obstructive lung, and inhibited healing.[5]

Several articles have suggested that the key to preventing prolonged air leaks is to assure the absence of leak intraoperatively by carefully testing staple lines for leaks under water, ensuring pleural apposition, and maintaining lung expansion.[9,16,18] However, in the case of patients undergoing lung volume reduction, this may not hold true. Many air leaks after LVRS are not present during or immediately after surgery, but develop some hours to days after the operation.[7,12] Date and colleagues[19] noted that 13% of patients undergoing LVRS developed a late air leak, attributed to sudden lung rupture in the postsurgical period. This finding may be the result of a redistribution of forces across the lung caused by newly created staple lines, which can form delayed tears in the fragile pleura of patients selected to undergo LVRS. These tears may even occur some distance away from the newly created staple lines.

There have been mixed outcomes from studying the use of buttressing materials, sealants, and glues in LVRS.[6,10,16,20] Staple line reinforcement may seal air leaks detected intraoperatively, but they also may redistribute forces across the lung and create tears and susbsequent air leaks remote from the line of resection as a result. Therefore, buttressing the staple line may have no effect in preventing the development of air leaks that develop after the operation.[12,20]

Another reason that patients undergoing LVRS may suffer prolonged air leaks relates to occult pulmonary comorbidities. In a study of 80 resection specimens of patients who underwent LVRS, Keller and colleagues[21] found numerous other unsuspected diagnoses in 37.5% of cases. Diagnoses included fibrosis, tumor, noncaseating granulomas, and infections, and patients who exhibited these in addition to their emphysema had significantly more complications. Patients with dual diagnoses had higher rates of prolonged air leak and needed significantly longer duration of tube thoracostomy and hospital stay. They had a higher rate of reintubation and reoperation for prolonged air leak.[21] Staple line stressors may be compounded by other lung abnormalities in patients exhibiting prolonged air leak. These factors may affect severely damaged lung parenchyma and cause bleb rupture.[20]

## NO-CUT PLICATION: DURABLE REDUCTION OF PROLONGED AIR LEAK?

If prolonged air leaks occur predominantly as a result of staple line stress, then avoiding staple lines should reduce the rate of prolonged air leak. This theory was tested by Crosa-Dorado and colleagues in a work published in 1992.[22] Swanson and colleagues[23] performed thoracoscopic no-cut plication in 50 operations on 32 patients with emphysema. Rate of prolonged air leak was found to be 9%, and atrial fibrillation rather than prolonged air leak was the most common complication in this group of LVRS patients. Additional benefits were seen in the cohort, including shorter hospital stay, lower mortality, and less need for intensive care unit (ICU) care and reintubation.[23] Iwasaki and colleagues[24] performed fold plication LVRS on 20 patients using a no-cut stapler. Air leaks subsided for all patients by postoperative day 5; however, 1 patient developed pneumothorax.[25] Mineo and colleagues[26] reported a 25% rate of prolonged air leak in 12 patients undergoing introflexion and plication with a no-knife stapler. Tacconi and colleagues[12] performed awake introflexion of lung apex with a noncutting staple applied to 3 short interrupted segments of apex on 66 patients between 2001 and 2008. A retrospective review of these prospectively collected data was compared with a historical control group of 66 patients. Prolonged air leak rate was found to be 40% in the traditional resection group, and 18% in the plicated group (Table 1).[12]

The results of these studies are encouraging, but many questions remain. Resected lung is permanently removed, and it has been speculated that the plicated segments may unfold in time. In most reported studies, the patient cohorts were followed for a period of months after surgery. Although gains in pulmonary function compare favorably with resection techniques, questions have arisen regarding the long-term durability of this technique. Pompeo and Mineo,[27] in a retrospective study, reported encouraging long-term results at 24 months of follow-up of their cohort of 12 patients. More long-term follow-up is warranted to evaluate for sustained improvements in pulmonary function after these techniques, perhaps in the form of a randomized trial comparing traditional resection with plication.

## RECENT EFFORTS TO REDUCE PROLONGED AIR LEAK IN LVRS

Two small randomized studies of LVRS patients raised the question of the benefit of fibrin sealants in reinforcing staple lines. Moser and colleagues,[28] from 2005 to 2006, randomized 22 patients in a study of the effect of reinforcing staple lines with an autologous fibrin sealant in LVRS on the incidence of prolonged air leak and duration of chest tube drainage. The sealant was made by transforming a sample of the patient's own blood into a sprayable, evenly coating fibrin sealant applied to a 1 cm margin around the interrupted staple lines. The rate of prolonged air leak in the sample treated with the fibrin sealant was 4.6%, significantly less than the rate of 32% seen in the nontreated group. The duration of chest tube drainage was also significantly lower (2.8 vs 5.9 days).[28]

Another randomized pilot study sought to compare BioGlue with bovine pericardium-buttressed staple lines. BioGlue is a sealant composed of bovine serum albumin and glutaraldehyde, packaged in an injectable syringe. Studies of glutaraldehyde-containing sealant showed promising results in animal models when used to seal staple lines of nonemphysematous lung. Ten patients undergoing resectional LVRS were randomly assigned to receive Peri-strips (staple line-reinforcing bovine pericardium) or Bio-Glue at the staple lines. The overall rate of prolonged air leak in this series of 10 patients was 50%, with 75% of these occurring in the pericardium-buttressed side.[29]

**Table 1**
Outcomes in patients undergoing no-cut plication for lung volume reduction

| Study | Unilateral Versus Bilateral | No. Patients | Months Follow-Up | Δ FEV1 (%) | Δ FVC (%) | Δ 6 min Walk Test (%) | % Prolonged Air Leak |
|---|---|---|---|---|---|---|---|
| Swanson et al, 1997[23] | Unilateral | 12 | 3.8±0.9 | ↑26 | ↑12±6 per side plicated | — | 9 combined rate |
|  | Bilateral | 10 | 5.1±0.9 | ↑55 |  | — | — |
| Kuwahira et al, 2000[25] | Unilateral | 20 | 6 | ↑31 | ↑11 | ↑20 | [a] |
| Mineo et al, 2006[26] | Unilateral | 12 | 6 | ↑31[b] | ↑19[b] | ↑19[b] | 25 |
|  | Unilateral | 12 | 24[c] | FEV1 stable | FVC stable | Stable | — |
| Tacconi et al, 2009[12] | Unilateral | 66 | 6 | ↑33[d] | ↑14[d] | ↑41[d] | 18[d] |

[a] Rate of prolonged air leak not reported, but the investigators did report a mean duration of chest tube drainage of 1.7 days, suggesting low rates of prolonged air leak.

[b] Calculated as a percentage change from pre- and postoperative FEV1, FVC, and 6 minute walk test.

[c] Twenty-four–month follow-up of the 12-patient cohort reported by Pompeo and Mineo (2007).[27]

[d] Calculated as a combined result of patients undergoing awake nonresectional surgery and nonresectional surgery under general anesthesia.

## PROLONGED AIR LEAK IN THE MECHANICALLY VENTILATED PATIENT

Potential complications of a prolonged air leak in mechanically ventilated patients include persistent pneumothorax, poor lung expansion from loss of tidal volume, ventilation-perfusion mismatch, infiltration of infection into the pleural space, inability to maintain positive expiratory end pressure (PEEP), and, ultimately, inability to adequately ventilate the patient, occasionally causing an insurmountable respiratory acidosis.[30]

Kempainen and Pierson[31] ascribed specific definitions to the various terms used to describe prolonged air leak in the diverse mechanically ventilated population. Air leak persisting for longer than 24 hours is termed a fistula. A bronchopleural fistula is an air leak that stems from a direct communication between main or segmental bronchi and the pleural cavity. A parenchymal-pleural fistula is an air leak from lung parenchyma, presumably at the alveolar level.[31]

## CAUSES OF AIR LEAK IN THE MECHANICALLY VENTILATED PATIENT

One way of gaining perspective on the characteristics of air leak in the population of mechanically ventilated patients is to study a sample of the ventilated population. In a prospective cohort study of 5183 patients receiving mechanical ventilation for more than 12 hours, representing 361 ICUs in 20 countries, in a 28-day period in 1998, Esteban and colleagues[32] reported an overall rate of barotraumas (air leak) of 3%. Patients were intubated for reasons that included postoperative respiratory failure (21%), coma (17%), pneumonia (14%), chronic obstructive pulmonary disease (COPD; 10%), congestive heart failure (10%), sepsis (9%), acquired respiratory distress syndrome (ARDS; 5%), aspiration (3%), asthma (2%), trauma (8%), and neuromuscular disease (2%). A subsequent study of barotrauma cases from this dataset revealed that 80% of patients presented with air leaks within 3 days of onset of mechanical ventilation.[32] However, a subset of patients developed air leaks more than 2 weeks after the onset of ventilation, most of whom had developed ARDS.[33]

In their seminal work on the subject of prolonged air leak in ventilated patients, Pierson and colleagues[30] reviewed 1700 mechanically ventilated patients, 39 (2%) of whom had bronchopleural fistulas that lasted more than 24 hours. They noted 3 processes that could lead to prolonged air leak in the ventilated patient: blunt or penetrating chest trauma, iatrogenic causes, and alveolar injury

stemming from ARDS. The overall mortality in their group of patients was 67%, and they noted significantly higher mortality among patients developing air leaks more than 24 hours after admission; patients developing pleural space infections; and those with a leak quantified at more than 500 mL per tidal volume.[30] A study of air leak in mechanically ventilated children noted different processes leading to high rates of air leak: congenital pulmonary disease (eg, Kartagener syndrome, deficiency of bronchial cartilage, right middle lobe syndrome, bronchiectasis), ARDS, and airway foreign bodies. This study showed that patients with documented infections and higher ventilatory flow rates had significantly more prolonged air leak.[34] Persistent air leaks in trauma patients most often seems to be caused by unhealed parenchymal injury,[35] but the cause of prolonged air leak is occasionally more complicated. Retained hemothorax or empyema, cavitation from penetrating trauma, and lung herniation at the site of penetrating rib fractures have been described.[36]

The finding of significantly higher mortality in ventilated patients who develop air leak has been echoed in several studies.[33,34,37] Patients who develop air leaks later in the course of mechanical ventilation have even higher mortality.[30] Early in the course of mechanical ventilation, gas is preferentially delivered to normal alveoli. Larger tidal volumes cause overdistention of alveoli, and high airway pressures can cause high shear stress on these alveoli, resulting in barotrauma or volutrauma and air leak. Later in the course of ventilation, derecruitment of alveoli at the junction of aerated and collapsed lung occurs. Ischemic or infective necrosis of persistently collapsed lung may occur, causing a second wave of air leak. Infection compounds the problem by recruiting leukocytes to the area and perpetuating the cycle of inflammatory mediators.[34,38] Chronic leukocyte sequestration causes mild emphysema due to repetitive release of leukocyte elastase, resulting in elastin degradation, airspace enlargement, and alveolar rupture.[34,39] Add to these the problems of malnutrition and multiple organ failure in the ventilated patient, and the reported high mortality is not surprising.

## MANAGEMENT OF PROLONGED AIR LEAKS IN VENTILATED PATIENTS

Regardless of the source of a persistent air leak, management strategies seem to be compatible, and are based on common principles. The wide adaptation of lung-protective ventilatory strategies has reduced the incidence of air leak in the ventilated population,[33] and is also the basis of management once it occurs.[40] Plateau airway pressures are a suitably accurate representation of transalveolar pressure, and reducing these to a value of less than 35 cm $H_2O$ is believed to be protective in lung injury patients.[10,11]

Suction applied to a thoracostomy tube can increase the volume of air leak across a fistula, inhibiting its healing and making ventilation difficult. Various chest tube management strategies have been examined in several randomized controlled studies in the postoperative setting.[42–46] The evidence favors water seal instead of suction in bringing about resolution of postoperative air leak. In cases of symptomatic or sizeable pneumothorax, a low level of suction (−10 cm water pressure) can be applied,[44] with early transition to water seal when feasible.[31]

## INTERVENTIONS TO ADDRESS PROLONGED AIR LEAK IN VENTILATED PATIENTS

Numerous novel endobronchial methods for addressing prolonged air leak have been documented.[47] Several studies have detailed varying levels of success with the use of sclerosants or sealants instilled through the thoracostomy tube and autologous blood patch pleurodesis for cessation of persistent air leak after pulmonary resection. None of these studies focused on the ventilated population per se, therefore the evidence to extend these therapies to mechanically ventilated patients does not exist. There is evidence that blood patch instillation leads to a higher rate of empyema.[31,48] Given that the causes of air leak in most ventilated patients stem from primary pulmonary conditions, acute lung injury (ALI)/ARDS or infection(s), instilling sealants or blood into the intrapleural space has its own attendant risks. Addressing the underlying illness and ventilator strategies designed to improve lung compliance seem to be the ultimate solutions to treating prolonged air leaks in this population.

There is a subset of patients with primary pulmonary diseases in whom air leak is so substantial that the patient cannot be adequately ventilated.[30] In these patients, extracorporeal membrane oxygenation (ECMO) may provide the only possible support. A recent randomized controlled trial assigned adults in severe respiratory failure to receive maximal conventional ventilatory therapy or ECMO. Ninety patients were assigned to each group. Intention-to-treat analysis revealed that ECMO-treated patients had better 6-month survival than conventionally ventilated patients. Limitations of the study include inconsistent conventional ventilation protocols and incomplete data for conventionally ventilated patients at 6 months. As expected, ECMO was expensive, with costs more than double those ascribed to conventionally ventilated patients.[49] However, in a patient with isolated severe respiratory failure in whom conventional methods of ventilation fail because of a large air leak, ECMO may be a viable, though expensive and morbid, means of supportive care that may be the only option for survival when available. As there is no documentation in the literature that ECMO has ever been used to bridge a patient through a ventilation-limiting air leak; it is at present a theoretical means of supportive care in these patients.

## SUMMARY

Prolonged air leak remains the biggest barrier to improving outcomes in patients undergoing LVRS. Because prolonged air leaks may develop some hours to days after the operation, they are different from air leaks that are seen intraoperatively and immediately postoperatively. Prolonged air leaks are probably caused by stresses and subsequent visceral pleural tears redistributed within the emphysematous lung that manifest at variable times during the postoperative course and at points distant from the staple line. Buttressing the staple line with bovine pericardium strips has no effect in reducing the rate of these prolonged air leaks, and may provoke morbid inflammatory reactions. Autologous fibrin sealants and BioGlue may have improved profiles of reducing prolonged air leak after LVRS. No-cut plication methods manifest the lowest rates of prolonged air leak in any LVRS, yet long-term data are limited.

Prolonged air leaks in the general ventilated population occur in a trimodal distribution. Traumatic pulmonary insults manifest air leak immediately on presentation. A subset of these trauma patients will develop prolonged air leak largely due to parenchymal injury. Air leak manifests at 2 to 3 days after the initiation of mechanical ventilation in patients with chronic interstitial lung disease, ALI/ARDS, and pneumonia. A third wave of air leak is seen after the first week of continuous mechanical ventilation, due largely to infectious complications in stressed and fragile lung parenchyma. All such patients require tube thoracostomy. Subsets of each category of patients will persist with air leak beyond 7 days. Lung-protective strategies have reduced the incidence of barotraumas/air leak and its duration in mechanically ventilated patients. Management of prolonged air leak in this population also includes minimizing volume escape by judicious chest tube management including minimal suction. Pleurodesis with chemicals, sealants, or autologous blood carry attendant risks given the high prevalence of coincident pulmonary infection. ECMO may be an alternative means of supportive care when the air leak is too large to permit adequate gas exchange through mechanical ventilation.

## REFERENCES

1. Brantigan OC, Mueller E, Kress MB. A surgical approach to pulmonary emphysema. Am Rev Respir Dis 1959;80:194–202.
2. Cooper JD, Patterson GA, Sundaresan RS, et al. Results of 150 consecutive bilateral lung volume reduction procedures in patients with severe emphysema. J Thorac Cardiovasc Surg 1996;112: 1319–30.
3. Criner GJ, O'Brien G, Furukawa S, et al. Lung volume reduction surgery in ventilator-dependent COPD patients. Chest 1996;110:877–84.
4. Cooper JD. The history of surgical procedures for emphysema. Ann Thorac Surg 1997;63:312–9.
5. DeCamp MM, Blackstone EH, Naunheim KS, et al. Patient and surgical factors influencing air leak after lung volume reduction surgery: lessons learned from the national emphysema treatment trial. Ann Thorac Surg 2006;82:197–207.
6. Stammberger U, Thurnheer R, Bloch KE, et al. Thoracoscopic bilateral lung volume reduction for diffuse pulmonary emphysema. Eur J Cardiothorac Surg 1997;11:1005–10.
7. McKenna RJ, Benditt JO, DeCamp MM, et al. Safety and efficacy of median sternotomy versus video-assisted thoracic surgery for lung volume reduction. J Thorac Cardiovasc Surg 2004;127: 1350–60.
8. Roberts JR, Bavaria JE, Wahl P, et al. Comparison of open and thoracoscopic bilateral volume reduction surgery: complications analysis. Ann Thorac Surg 1998;66:1759–65.
9. Cooper JD. Technique to reduce air leaks after resection of emphysematous lung. Ann Thorac Surg 1994;57:1038–9.
10. Stammberger U, Klepetko W, Stamatis G, et al. Buttressing the staple line in lung volume reduction surgery: a randomized three-center study. Ann Thorac Surg 2000;70:1820–5.
11. Tiong LU, Gibson PG, Hensley MJ, et al. Lung volume reduction surgery for diffuse emphysema. Cochrane Database Syst Rev 2006;4:CD001001.
12. Tacconi F, Pompeo E, Mineo TC. Duration of air leak is reduced after awake nonresectional lung volume reduction surgery. Eur J Cardiothorac Surg 2009; 35:822–8.
13. Provencher S, Deslauriers J. Late complication of bovine pericardium patches used for lung volume reduction surgery. Eur J Cardiothorac Surg 2003; 23(6):1059–61.
14. McKenna RJ, Brenner M, Gelb AF, et al. A randomized, prospective trial of stapled lung reduction vs laser bullectomy for diffuse emphysema. J Thorac Cardiovasc Surg 1996;111(2):293–5.
15. Busetto A, Moretti R, Barbaresco S, et al. Extrapleural bullectomy or lung volume reduction: air tight surgery for emphysema without strip-patch. Acta Chir Hung 1999;38(1):15–7.
16. Toloza EM, Harpole DH. Intraoperative techniques to prevent air leaks. Chest Surg Clin N Am 2002;12: 489–505.
17. Brunelli A, Monteverde M, Borri A, et al. Predictors of prolonged air leak after pulmonary lobectomy. Ann Thorac Surg 2004;77:1205–10.
18. Rice TW, Okereke IC, Blackstone EH. Persistent airleak following pulmonary resection. Chest Surg Clin N Am 2002;12:529–39.
19. Date H, Goto K, Souda R, et al. Bilateral lung volume reduction surgery via median sternotomy for severe pulmonary emphysema. Ann Thorac Surg 1998;65: 939–42.
20. Fischel RJ, McKenna RJ. Bovine pericardium versus bovine collagen to buttress staples for lung reduction operations. Ann Thorac Surg 1998;65:217–9.
21. Keller CA, Naunheim KS, Osterloh J, et al. Histopathologic diagnosis made in lung tissue resected from patients with severe emphysema undergoing lung volume reduction surgery. Chest 1997;111:941–7.
22. Crosa-Dorado VL, Pomi J, Perez-Penco EJ, et al. Treatment of dyspnea in emphysema: pulmonary remodelling. Hemo- and pneumostatic suturing of the emphysematous lung. Research in Surgery 1992; 4(3):1–4.
23. Swanson SJ, Mentzer SJ, DeCamp MM, et al. No-cut thoracoscopic lung plication: a new technique for lung volume reduction surgery. J Am Coll Surg 1997;185:25–32.
24. Iwasaki M, Nishiumi N, Kaga K, et al. Application of the fold plication method for unilateral lung volume reduction on pulmonary emphysema. Ann Thorac Surg 1999;67:815–7.
25. Kuwahira I, Iwasaki M, Kaga K, et al. Effectiveness of the fold plication method in lung volume reduction surgery. Intern Med 2000;39(5):381–4.
26. Mineo TC, Pompeo E, Mineo D, et al. Awake nonresectional lung volume reduction surgery. Ann Surg 2006;243:131–6.
27. Pompeo E, Mineo TC. Two-year improvement in multidimensional body mass index, airflow obstruction, dyspnea, and exercise capacity index after nonresectional lung volume reduction surgery in awake patients. Ann Thorac Surg 2007;84:1862–9.
28. Moser C, Opitz I, Zhai W, et al. Autologous fibrin sealant reduces the incidence of prolonged air leak and duration of chest tube drainage after lung

volume reduction surgery: a prospective random-ized blinded study. J Thorac Cardiovasc Surg 2008;136:843–9.

29. Rathinam S, Naidu BV, Nanjaiah P, et al. BioGlue and Peri-strips in lung volume reduction surgery: pilot randomised controlled trial. J Cardiothorac Surg 2009;4:37–42.

30. Pierson DJ, Horton CA, Bates PW. Persistent bron-chopleural air leak during mechanical ventilation. Chest 1986;90:321–3.

31. Kempainen RR, Pierson DJ. Persistent air leaks in patients receiving mechanical ventilation. Semin Re-spir Crit Care Med 2001;22(6):675–84.

32. Esteban AE, Anzueto A, Frutos F, et al. Charac-teristics and outcomes in adult patients receiving mechanical ventilation. JAMA 2002; 287:345–55.

33. Anzueto A, Frutos-Vivar F, Esteban A, et al. Inci-dence, risk factors and outcome of barotrauma in mechanically ventilated patients. Intensive Care Med 2004;30:612–9.

34. Briassoulis GC, Venkataraman ST, Vasilopoulos AG, et al. Air leaks from the respiratory tract in mechan-ically ventilated children with severe respiratory disease. Pediatr Pulmonol 2000;29:127–34.

35. Schermer CR, Matteson BD, Demarest GB, et al. A prospective evaluation of video-assisted thoracic surgery for persistent air leak due to trauma. Am J Surg 1999;177:480–4.

36. Carillo EH, Schmacht DC, Gable DR, et al. Thora-coscopy in the management of posttraumatic persistent pneumothorax. J Am Coll Surg 1998; 186:636–40.

37. Brun-Buisson C, Minelli C, Bertolini G, et al. Epide-miology and outcome of acute lung injury in Euro-pean intensive care units. Intensive Care Med 2004;30:51–61.

38. Reimel BA, Krishnadasen B, Cuschieri J, et al. Surgical management of acute necrotizing lung infections. Can Respir J 2006;13(7):369–73.

39. Parsons PE, Eisner MD, Thompson BT, et al. Lower tidal volume ventilation and plasma cytokine markers of inflammation in patients with acute lung injury. Crit Care Med 2005;33:1–6.

40. Cho MH, Malhotra A, Donahue DM, et al. Mechan-ical ventilation and air leaks after lung biopsy for acute respiratory distress syndrome. Ann Thorac Surg 2006;82:261–6.

41. Brochard L, Roudot-Thoraval F, Roupie E, et al. Tidal volume reduction for prevention of ventilator-induced lung injury in acute respiratory distress syndrome. The Multicenter Trial Group on tidal volume reduction in ARDS. Am J Respir Crit Care Med 1998;158(6):1831–8.

42. Cerfolio RJ, Bass CS, Katholi CR, et al. Prospective randomized trial compares suction versus water seal for air leaks. Ann Thorac Surg 2001;71:1613–7.

43. Marshall MB, Deeb ME, Bleier JI, et al. Suction vs water seal after pulmonary resection. A randomized prospective study. Chest 2002;121:831–5.

44. Brunelli A, Sabbatini A, Xiume F, et al. Alternate suction reduces prolonged air leak after pulmonary lobectomy: a randomized comparison versus water seal. Ann Thorac Surg 2005;80:1052–5.

45. Alphonso N, Tan C, Utley M, et al. A prospective randomized controlled trial of suction versus non-suction to the under-water seal drains following lung resection. Eur J Cardiothorac Surg 2005;27:391–4.

46. Cerfolio RJ. Recent advances in the treatment of air leaks. Curr Opin Pulm Med 2005;11(4):319–23.

47. Travaline JM, McKenna RJ, De Giacomo T, et al. Treatment of persistent pulmonary air leaks using endobronchial valves. Chest 2009;136:355–60.

48. Shackcloth MJ, Poullis M, Jackson M, et al. Intra-pleural instillation of autologous blood in the treat-ment of prolonged air leak after lobectomy: a prospective randomized controlled trial. Ann Thor-ac Surg 2006;82:1052–6.

49. Peek GJ, Mugford M, Tiruvaipathi R, et al. Efficacy and economic assessment of conventional ventila-tory support versus extracorporeal membrane oxygenation for severe adult respiratory failure (CE-SAR): a multicentre randomised controlled trial. Lancet 2009;374:1351–63.

# Evidence-Based Suggestions for Management of Air Leaks

Robert E. Merritt, MD[a],*, Sunil Singhal, MD[b],
Joseph B. Shrager, MD[a,c]

## KEYWORDS

- Air leak • Alveolar air leak • Thoracostomy
- Pneumothorax • Bronchopleural fistula • Emphysema
- Stapling devices • Pulmonary lobectomy

Alveolar air leaks (AALs) that occur after pulmonary resection are a significant clinical problem in the practice of thoracic surgery. AALs that persist beyond the immediate postoperative period are associated with a variety of complications, and they can result in increased hospital length of stay (LOS) and increased costs. Many studies have been published in recent years to evaluate the products and techniques designed to prevent or ameliorate AALs. Many of the methods proposed to minimize postoperative AALs add substantial cost to the operations for which they might be used, and therefore deserve careful scrutiny. This article presents an evidenced-based review of all of the available literature to determine which approaches to the problem of AALs have the greatest scientific support.

During the initial management of a postoperative AALs, the surgeon generally does not know whether such a leak originates from the alveoli via a peripheral tear in the visceral pleura (ie, an AAL) or whether it originates from bronchial structures (ie, a bronchopleural fistula [BPF]). Most postoperative AALs will ultimately prove to be AALs; therefore, the initial management should be aimed at treating an AAL. However, leakage of air that is ultimately proven to be a BPF is managed differently from an AAL, often requiring early surgical intervention, and this topic is not discussed in detail within this article.

## THE CONCEPT OF PROLONGED AIR LEAK

The many published studies that have addressed AALs have used several different definitions for the term prolonged air leak (PAL); from an AAL lasting 4 days postoperatively to one lasting more than 10 days postoperatively. Perhaps the major impetus to labeling an AAL a PAL is related to postoperative LOS. An AAL can be considered to be a PAL when the leakage of air, and the resulting need for chest tube drainage, is the only problem requiring a patient to remain in the hospital. At this point, placement of a Heimlich valve might be considered. Because recent studies of pulmonary lobectomy have recorded mean LOS in the 5-day range, the authors suggest that a modern definition of a PAL should be a leak lasting beyond postoperative day (POD) 5.

The authors have nothing to disclose.

[a] Division of Thoracic Surgery, Department of Cardiothoracic Surgery, Stanford University School of Medicine, Stanford Medical Center, 2nd floor Falk Building, 300 Pasteur Drive, Stanford, CA 94305, USA
[b] Division of Thoracic Surgery, Hospital of the University of Pennsylvania, University of Pennsylvania School of Medicine, 6th floor Ravdin Building, 3400 Spruce Street, Philadelphia, PA 19104, USA
[c] Veterans Affairs Palo Alto Health Care System, Building 100, Room F4-210, 3801 Miranda Avenue, Palo Alto, CA 94304, USA
* Corresponding author.
E-mail address: rmerritt@stanford.edu

# INCIDENCE, SIGNIFICANCE, AND RISK FACTORS FOR AIR LEAKS

## Incidence of Air Leak

The presence or absence of AAL has been recorded at different postoperative time points in different studies. Immediately at the completion of surgery, AAL has been reported to be present in between 28% and 60%[1–5] of patients having routine pulmonary resection reported in series that included lobectomies and lesser resections. On the morning of POD1, an AAL is present in 26% to 48% of patients,[6,7] and on the morning of POD2 AAL is present in 22% to 24% of cases.[6,8] On the morning of POD4, AALs were present in one study in 8% of cases.[9] In the lung volume reduction surgery (LVRS) population, AAL occurred at some point during the postoperative period in 90% of patients undergoing bilateral procedures within the National Emphysema Treatment Trial (NETT).[10]

## Incidence of PAL

Although PAL is defined variably, its incidence has been reported to be present in 8% to 26%[9,11,12] of patients undergoing routine pulmonary resections. Following LVRS in the NETT, the median duration of air leak (AL) was 7 days, and 12% of patients had a persistent AL even at 30 days postoperatively.[10] In patients with forced expiratory volume in 1 second ($FEV_1$) less than 35% predicted undergoing non-LVRS unilateral pulmonary resections, 22% had an AL lasting more than 7 days.[13] In the population of patients undergoing lung biopsy for interstitial lung disease (ILD), PAL has been reported to occur in 1.6% to 30.2% of patients,[14–16] clearly related to whether the patients being reported are outpatients with mild disease or inpatients requiring mechanical ventilation for severe disease.

## Significance of AL/PAL

Several studies have found that PAL increases complication rates after routine pulmonary resection. Empyema[17] and other pulmonary complications[18] have been associated with PAL. Okereke and colleagues[4] found that any AL was associated with more complications (30% vs 18%, $P = .07$). This finding was also true in the LVRS population (57% vs 30%, $P = .0004$).[10] In one study of 53 patients with acute respiratory distress syndrome (ARDS) who required lung biopsy, there was a trend toward higher mortality in patients with PAL.[16]

It has also been shown in many studies that PAL increases LOS and costs. Every study in the routine lung resection population reporting LOS or costs as a function of PAL has found an association. Varela and colleagues[11] found LOS to be increased by about 6 days at a total expense of more than 39,000 euros. Brunelli and colleagues[17] found LOS to be increased by 7.9 days. Bardell and Petsikas[12] found that, of all factors studied, only PAL was predictive of increased LOS. Irshad and colleagues[18] found that the 3 most frequent complications that delayed discharge beyond POD5 were PAL, pulmonary infection, and atrial fibrillation; PAL increased LOS by a mean of 13.1 days. In the LVRS population,[10] the mean LOS among survivors was 11.8 days in those with any AAL versus 7.6 days in those without AAL ($P = .0005$).

## Risk Factors for AL/PAL

The most consistently identified risk factor for PAL is chronic obstructive pulmonary disease (COPD). Many of the various preoperative tests that reflect severity of COPD have been associated with PAL.[9,12,19,20] Patients with severe emphysema who require LVRS are especially susceptible to PAL,[10] as are those with $FEV_1$ less than 35% predicted who require other types of pulmonary resections.[13] There is clearly a strong positive correlation between degree of emphysema and risk of AAL and PAL.

Other important risk factors associated with PAL in 1 or more studies include presence of adhesions,[19] upper lobectomy and bilobectomy,[19] lobectomy versus lesser resections,[9] presence of a pneumothorax coinciding with the AAL,[9,21] steroid use greater than 10 mg daily for more than 1 month,[9] and a leak of a size greater than 4 on the scale of 1 to 7 proposed by Cerfolio and colleagues.[9] In a retrospective study of intubated patients undergoing lung biopsy for ARDS, the only multivariate predictor of PAL was peak airway pressure (PAP). The risk of PAL was reduced by 42% for every 5 cm $H_2O$ reduction in PAP. A lower risk of AL was associated with lower PAP, lower tidal volume, and use of pressure-cycled ventilation.[16]

## Grading System for ALs

Cerfolio and colleagues[8] described a useful semiquantitative classification of ALs. Using the airleak meter that is part of the Pleur-evac system (Deknatel, Boston, MA, USA), AALs were scored on a scale of 1 to 7 according to the highest-numbered chamber reached by bubbles with deep breathing or coughing (for a leak present only on coughing). The largest number consistently reached was the number assigned. Interobserver variability was reasonably good.

In this single institution, this scoring system has proven to have prognostic value. First, in protocols that assayed the use of waterseal to reduce duration of AAL, every patient who developed a pneumothorax when placed on waterseal had a leak that was at least 4/7 on the scale, and a leak of this size predicted a PAL ($P<.001$). All patients whose leaks stopped when placed on waterseal had a leak of 3/7 or less.[8] A leak 4/7 or greater was also found to be highly predictive of failure of waterseal in patients with AL and pneumothorax.[21] Clearly, patients with a leak 4/7 or greater are not ideal candidates to place on waterseal. However, this grading system needs to be confirmed in other institutions.

Several published studies have performed initial evaluations of products designed to quantitatively measure ALs using digital technology. Three of these are randomized studies.[22–24] Although these digital AL measurement devices do seem to provide more detailed and consistent AL data, it is not clear that they provide sufficiently improved decision making regarding timing of chest tube removal to justify their increased cost.

## INTRAOPERATIVE MANAGEMENT OF ALs

Postoperative AALs may occur directly at staple lines, from tissues adjacent to staple lines, from sites where pleural adhesions have been taken down, and from areas of dissection such as within fissures and around lymph nodes. The optimal time to manage these AALs is intraoperatively. Beyond simply resuturing the areas of visible AL, several other intraoperative techniques have been introduced to try to reduce postoperative AALs. The 2 most recent techniques introduced are buttressing the staple line and using sealing agents to close leaks from visceral pleural breaches. Other more traditional alternatives include pleural tenting and the creation of a pneumoperitoneum.

Cooper[25] first reported the use of bovine pericardium in buttressing staple lines to control ALs following LVRS. Subsequently, several researchers have supported the use of bovine pericardium to control ALs, not only in patients with emphysema but also in patients without emphysema undergoing pulmonary resection.[26] Many other materials are also used as buttresses, including excised parietal pleura, polydioxane ribbon, Teflon felt, expanded polytetrafluoroethylene, and collagen patches.[27] Nonabsorbable materials carry the risk of inducing granulomatous inflammation and bacterial colonization, which has even led in some cases to metalloptysis. This event has been described in several case reports, largely with the use of bovine pericardium. Four randomized studies compared buttressed to nonbuttressed stapling of resection lines, 2 in patients having LVRS[28,29] and 2 in patients having lobectomy.[30,31]

### Buttressing Staple Lines in Patients Who are not Severely Emphysematous

Two randomized studies in patients undergoing pulmonary resection predominately for lung cancer evaluated bovine pericardium for staple line reinforcement. Venuta and colleagues[31] (n = 30) found decreased AALs and shorter hospital stay, whereas Miller and colleagues[30] (n = 80) found reduced duration of AAL but no significant difference in LOS. In the study by Venuta and colleagues,[31] fissures were completed with gastrointestinal anastomosis (GIA) staplers buttressed with bovine pericardial sleeves (n = 10), TA 55 staplers alone (n = 10), or clamps and silk ties (n = 10). Postoperative AALs persisted for 2 days in the group with buttressed staple lines compared with 5 days in the other 2 groups. Mean LOS was significantly shorter at 4 days compared with 7 days in the nonbuttressed resections ($P$ = .0001). The lack of the ideal control group using unbuttressed GIA staplers and the small numbers in this study limits the conclusions that can be drawn from it.

Miller and colleagues[30] performed a multicenter trial consisting of 80 patients undergoing pulmonary resection, randomly assigned to the unbuttressed control group or staple line reinforcement with bovine pericardium. Increased AAL duration was associated with assignment to the control group (r = 0.27, $P$ = .02), but there were no statistical differences in the mean intensive care unit LOS ($P$ = .9), number of days with a chest drain ($P$ = .6), or total LOS ($P$ = .24).

Although both of these studies of buttressing staple lines in patients without severe COPD suggest that buttressing slightly reduces duration of AALs, the larger and better-controlled trial did not identify a clear benefit of staple line reinforcement in terms of LOS or chest tube duration. Buttressing staples lines does add as much as several hundred dollars to hospital costs. Given the increased costs and unclear benefits, buttressing staple lines during pulmonary resection is not currently recommended for most patients with less than moderate emphysema.

### Buttressing Staple Lines in Patients with Severe Emphysema

Management of AALs is particularly challenging in patients having LVRS. DeCamp and colleagues[10] reviewed the entire population that underwent

LVRS in the NETT and found no benefit of using buttressed staple lines to prevent AALs. However, this analysis was not randomized on the basis of buttressing. Other groups have observed a benefit of reinforcing the staple line in patients with emphysema having LVRS. Two randomized clinical trials in this patient population found a benefit from buttressing staple lines.[28,29] A randomized 2-center study by Hazelrigg and colleagues[28] involving 123 patients undergoing unilateral thoracoscopic LVRS showed a significant decrease in the duration of postoperative ALs, earlier chest drain removal, and a shorter hospital stay in patients receiving bovine pericardial strips compared with patients without such buttressing. Costs were unchanged, because the costs of the pericardial sleeves offset the savings in hospital days. Stammberger and colleagues[29] presented a randomized 3-center study evaluating buttressing in LVRS. Sixty-five patients underwent bilateral LVRS by video-assisted thoracoscopy using endoscopic staplers, with or without bovine pericardium for buttressing. There was a significant decrease in the incidence of initial AAL: 77% versus 39%. Seven patients (3 in the treatment group) needed a reoperation because of persistent AAL. The median duration of AALs was shorter in the treatment group (0 vs 4 days; $P<.001$), and there was a shorter median drainage time in this group (5 vs 7.5 days; $P = .045$). Hospital stay was comparable between the 2 groups (9.5 vs 12.0 days; $P = .14$).

The evidence from randomized studies suggests that using buttresses on staple lines in patients with emphysema reduces the incidence of AALs when performing nonanatomic pulmonary resections such as LVRS. This technique permits the earlier removal of chest drains and shortens LOS. The use of buttresses in this population seems to be cost-neutral. The authors therefore believe that buttresses should be used in this scenario.

The high-quality data on buttressing staple lines in patients with emphysema come from the LVRS population that undergoes nonanatomic stapling (ie, wedge resection). There are insufficient data to support the routine use of staple line buttresses even in patients with severe emphysema when performing anatomic lobectomy or segmentectomy. However, the investigators believe that the benefit of buttressing staple lines in patients with severe emphysema likely translates to situations in which one is stapling incomplete interlobar fissures or intersegmental planes in patients with emphysema.

## Use of Topical Sealants

A variety of surgical sealants have been developed in an effort to prevent AALs. They are applied during operation over lung surfaces where violation of the visceral pleura has occurred. The sealants used include fibrin glues, synthetic polyethylene glycol–based hydrogel sealants, and fleece-bound sealants. Surgical sealants can be effective in reducing the percentage of patients who have a visible AAL at the conclusion of an operation. However, their overall benefit has not been established. Studies do not consistently show that sealants: (a) reduce the time to removal of chest drains, (b) decrease the LOS, or (c) reduce the duration of PAL.

Serra-Mitjans and colleagues[32] and Tambiah and colleagues[33] performed comprehensive reviews of the literature evaluating sealants to prevent AAL after pulmonary resections in patients with lung cancer. These reports identified several published and unpublished trials in which standard closure techniques plus a sealant were compared with the same intervention without a sealant. The outcomes measured included morbidity (AAL, wound infection, empyema), mortality, postoperative chest drain time, and postoperative hospital time. The 2005 report from Serra-Mitjans and colleagues[32] identified 12 randomized controlled trials with a total of 1097 patients, and **Table 1** incorporates an additional 4 randomized studies published since that time.

These studies describe many sealants following pulmonary resections. Fibrin glue, a sealant that consists of fibrinogen, factor XIII, fibronectin, aprotinin, plasminogen, and a thrombin solution, was evaluated in 6 trials.[34–38] A synthetic sealant consisting of polyethylene glycol, trimethylene carbonate, and acrylate was used in 2 trials.[39,40] A water-soluble polyethylene glycol–based gel photopolymerizable was used in 1 trial.[41] A polymeric biodegradable sealant (polyethylene glycol–based cross-linker, functionalized with succinate groups [PEG-(SS)2] with human serum albumin-USP [United States Pharmacopeia]) was used in 1 trial and a different polymeric sealant with used in another similar report.[42,43] TachoComb, an absorbable patch consisting of an equine-collagen fleece coated with human fibrinogen and human thrombin, was used in 1 study.[44] A slightly different human fibrinogen and thrombin mix (TachoSil) was used in 3 other reports.[45–47] Vivostat is an autologous fibrin sealant that was evaluated in 2 trials.[48,49] Tansley and colleagues[50] used a mixture of bovine serum albumin and glutaraldehyde (BioGlue) in a prospective, randomized trial of efficacy in treating AAL. The various sealants differ in how they are applied: aerosolized spraying mechanism, double syringe (with or without photopolymerization by xenon light), or a direct application of an absorbable patch.

**Table 1**
**Randomized controlled trials evaluating surgical sealants for intraoperative ALs**

| Author | Sealant | N | Patients with Postoperative ALs | Duration of AL | Duration of Chest Drain | Hospital Days |
|---|---|---|---|---|---|---|
| Allen et al[42] | Novel polymeric sealant | 148 | a | | | a |
| Belboul et al[48] | Visostat | 40 | a | | | |
| Fabian et al[34] | Fibrin glue | 100 | a | a | a | |
| Fleisher et al[35] | Fibrin glue | 28 | | | | |
| Lang et al[44] | TachoComb | 189 | a | | | |
| Macchiarini et al[40] | Fibrin glue | 26 | a | | | |
| Moser et al[49] | Fibrin glue | 25 (bilateral) | a | a | a | |
| Mouritzen et al[37] | Fibrin glue | 114 | a | | | a |
| Porte et al[39] | Advaseal | 120 | a | a | | |
| Tansley et al[50] | Bioglue | 52 | a | a | a | a |
| Wain et al[41] | FocalSeal | 172 | a | a | | |
| Wong and Goldstraw[36] | Fibrin glue | 66 | | | | |
| Wurtz et al[38] | Fibrin glue | 50 | a | | | |
| Wurtz et al[43] | Fibrin glue | 50 | a | | | |
| Anegg et al[47] | Fleece-bound sealing | 173 | a | a | a | a |
| D'Andrilli et al[45] | Polymeric sealant | 203 | a | a | | |

[a] Significant improvement in treated group versus untreated group. The empty cells indicate no significant difference or a variable that was not assessed.

Serra-Mitjans and colleagues[32] determined that the quality and methodology in these trials were variable. In most of the trials, there was no standard definition of AAL. In addition, the investigators made no attempt to quantify the degree of AAL in the perioperative period. In 3 trials, patients were randomized after checking for the presence of intraoperative AAL. In 9 of trials, the staple lines and cut surfaces of the lung parenchyma in the experimental group were routinely covered with topical sealant regardless of the presence of AAL.

In 11 trials, a significantly lower percentage of patients had AAL at the conclusion of the operation when sealants were used. However, Serra-Mitjans and colleagues[32] and Tambiah and colleagues[33] each point out that many of these trials do not show a reduction in number of chest tube days with the use of sealants. The limiting factor in removing chest drains in these patients was often the volume of fluid drainage rather than the presence or absence of AAL. There are only 3 studies with sealants that show a reduction in the number of chest tube days. Fabian and colleagues[34] found mean time to chest drain removal in the treatment group was 3.5 days and in the control group was 5 days. Tansley and colleagues[50] reported that patients who were treated with BioGlue had significantly shorter median duration of chest drainage; 4 versus 5 days ($P = .012$). More recently, Anegg and colleagues[47] attempted to seal grade 1 to 2 AALs visualized in the operating room with a fleece-bound collagen product (TachoSil) after routine fissure management. These results also showed significantly reduced number of chest tube days with the product ($P<.02$).

Hospital LOS has also not been generally reduced by topical sealants, although there is some evidence that this may occur. Allen and colleagues[42] found that the LOS was significantly reduced in the treatment group, but there was no reduction in time of chest drain duration. This seemingly contradictory result may be related to the use of Heimlich valves. This study also failed to show a reduction in the incidence of AAL requiring Heimlich valve in the sealant group. The

Tansley and colleagues[50] study of BioGlue showed a shorter median LOS; 6 versus 7 days ($P = .004$), compared with controls.

In patients who had an AAL postoperatively, regardless of whether a surgical sealant was used, there was a reduction in mean AAL duration time in 4 of the trials. ALs in the trial by Porte and colleagues[39] lasted a mean 33.70 hours in the treatment group and 63.22 hours in control group, and 30.90 hours and 52.30 hours respectively in the trial by Wain and colleagues.[41] ALs lasted a mean of 1.1 and 3.1 days in the treatment versus control group (respectively) in the trial by Fabian and colleagues.[34] In that trial there was a significantly higher rate of prolonged AALs in those patients who were not treated by sealants (2% vs 16%, $P = .015$). D'Andrilli and colleagues[45] described a randomized study to evaluate a polymeric sealant (CoSeal) in 203 patients with moderate/severe intraoperative ALs after anatomic pulmonary resections (n = 110) or minor resections (n = 93). Patients were randomly assigned to suture/stapling or suture/stapling plus CoSeal sealant. AL rates at 24 hours and 48 hours were significantly lower in the CoSeal group (19.6% vs 40.6%, $P = .001$ at 24 hours; 23.5% vs 41.6%, $P = .006$ at 48 hours) and the duration of ALs was significantly shorter in the CoSeal group ($P = .01$).

None of the randomized studies discussed earlier performed a subgroup analysis to evaluate the effectiveness of sealants in AAL of differing sizes. Similarly, none of these studies were targeted to patients who are at highest risk for complicated or prolonged AALs (ie, those with severe emphysema) or reported results in subgroups of patients with severe emphysema. Therefore, there is insufficient information currently available to determine whether there are specific subgroups of patients who more clearly benefit from the use of surgical sealants. There is 1 small randomized report of sealants in patients with severe emphysema, but in the LVRS setting. This report is of a prospective, randomized, blinded, sealant study in 25 patients undergoing bilateral thoracoscopic LVRS.[49] In each patient, an autologous fibrin sealant was applied along the staple line on 1 side of the chest only. The incidence of prolonged AALs and mean duration of drainage were significantly reduced on the sealant side (4.5% and 2.8 days vs 31.8% and 5.9 days).

Beyond the use of sealants after traditional parenchymal stapling, there have been recent reports that a particular type of sealant combined with electrocautery dissection of fissures may be superior to the use of stapler devices to divide fissures. Rena and colleagues[46] conducted a randomized trial of 60 patients with COPD ($FEV_1 < 65\%$) and fused fissures and reported that collagen patches coated with human fibrinogen and thrombin (TachoSil) following electrocautery dissection is more effective than stapling fissures in terms of length of chest tube drainage (mean 3.5 vs 5.9 days, $P = .0021$) and LOS (5.9 vs 7.5 days; $P = .01$). Another study randomized 40 patients to stapler dissection versus electrocautery dissection plus collagen patches coated with fibrinogen and thrombin.[45] In this study, there was a reduction in the duration of AALs in the electrocautery plus collagen group (1.7 vs 4.5 days, $P = .003$). This approach may prove to be more advantageous economically than adding sealants to standard staplers because it has the advantage of eliminating the costs of the staplers.

Most of the sealants studied seem to reduce the percentage of patients with a visible AAL at the end of an operative procedure. However, most of these sealants do not seem to alter the mean duration of AAL or mean duration of chest tube drainage to a clinically significant degree. Only 4 of 16 randomized studies show significantly reduced LOS in the sealant group, and only 2 studies (of BioGlue and TachoSil), clearly show the reduced AL duration and chest tube duration that would be expected to result in this reduced LOS. Almost none of the studies report on whether the sealants reduce complicated or prolonged AAL; the outcome variable that is perhaps most important to practicing surgeons. In addition, only 1 study of a liquid sealant applied the product to the highest risk group; those with substantial emphysema. This study showed a benefit to its sealant (autologous fibrin), suggesting that perhaps the sealants (like buttresses) might be appropriately applied to a select group of patients with substantial emphysema. Further study is required to determine whether that is appropriate.

Given the inconclusive results of sealant studies, and the significantly increased costs that would be incurred by using sealants indiscriminately, it is appropriate to use sealants only selectively at this point.

### Use of Pleural Tent

The creation of a pleural tent may eliminate an apical pleural space and facilitate the sealing of ALs. The predominant risk of this procedure is the development of a hemothorax. Most studies measure this complication by the need for postoperative blood transfusions. Three studies (2 randomized, 1 retrospective) evaluate this technique.

Brunelli and colleagues[51] performed a randomized prospective trial of pleural tents in patients undergoing upper lobectomy. Two hundred patients were prospectively randomized to tent or no tent. Pleural tent resulted in a significant reduction in the mean duration of AL (2.5 vs 7.2 days; P<0001), the number of days a chest drain was required (7.0 vs 11.2; P<.0001), and the LOS in days (8.2 vs 11.6; P<.0001). Multivariate analysis found that failure to have a pleural tent was an independent predictor of the occurrence and duration of AL. There was no increased need for blood transfusions in the pleural tent population.

Okur and colleagues[52] performed a prospective randomized study of pleural tent in 40 patients having upper or upper and middle lobectomies. Duration of chest drain drainage was shorter in the pleural tent group (4.3 ± 0.16 days vs 7.40 ± 0.68 days, P<.0001), as was mean LOS (7.60 ± 0.4 days vs 9.35 ± 0.6 days, P = .024). There was no significant difference in total pleural drainage volume between the groups. Three of 20 (15%) patients in the nontented group needed an apical chest drain insertion in the postoperative period for PAL with an apical space. Asymptomatic apical residual space occurred in 3 of 20 patients in the tented group. There was no morbidity in the patients in the tented group.

Robinson and colleagues[53] performed a retrospective study of 48 consecutive patients undergoing isolated upper lobectomy for neoplasm. In 3 years, 28 patients had creation of a pleural tent and 20 patients did not. Chest drains were removed according to a fixed protocol. The patients who were tented had significantly shorter mean AL duration (tented 1.6 ± 0.3 days vs nontented 3.9 ± 1.2 days, P = .04), mean total fluid drainage (tented 1619.5 ± 95.5 mL vs nontented 2476.3 ± 346.4 mL, P = .009), mean chest drain duration (tented 4.0 ± 0.2 days vs nontented 6.6 ± 1.0 days, P = .004), and mean LOS (tented 6.4 ± 0.4 days vs nontented 8.6 ± 1.0 days, P = .02). No operative deaths occurred, and morbidity was not significantly different between groups.

Pleural tenting therefore clearly reduces the duration of AL, the duration of chest drainage, and the LOS in patients undergoing upper lobectomy and upper bilobectomy, and it seems to incur little morbidity. It is therefore reasonable to use pleural tenting in combination with these resections. Subset analysis of patients with greater risk factors for the development of AL or PAL (eg, patients with more severe emphysema) was not performed in the studies of pleural tenting. The authors therefore are unable to determine whether there are specific subgroups of patients who derive the greatest benefit from pleural tenting. However, common sense suggests that tenting is more likely to be of most benefit in patients with moderate to severe emphysema.

### Use of Intraoperative Pneumoperitoneum

Toker and colleagues[54] examined the effectiveness of intraoperative pneumoperitoneum to reduce AAL after a lower lobectomy or lower bilobectomy for lung cancer. They studied 50 nonrandomized patients whose remnant lung failed to fill at least half of the hemithorax under positive pressure ventilation. Pneumoperitoneum significantly reduced the duration of postoperative AL (2.2 vs 6.0 days, P<.0001) and total chest drainage time (3.8 vs 7.9 days, P<.001).

Cerfolio and colleagues[55] presented data on creating a pneumoperitoneum in patients following removal of the right middle and lower lobes. They prospectively randomized 16 patients who underwent bilobectomy: 8 patients had 1200 mL of air injected through the right hemidiaphragm at the time of surgery and 8 did not. On POD1, AAL was present in 1 patient (13%) in the pneumoperitoneum group and 5 patients (63%) in the control group (P<.001). By POD3, 0% versus 50% had leaks, respectively (P<.001). Median hospital stay in the pneumoperitoneum group was 4 days compared with 6 days in the control group (P<.001). Three patients in the control group were discharged with a Heimlich valve. There were no complications related to the pneumoperitoneum.

Thus, although little published data exists, it seems likely that intraoperative creation of pneumoperitoneum reduces AL duration and LOS following lower lobectomy or lower bilobectomy. Again, subset analysis was not performed in the studies of pneumoperitoneum. The authors therefore do not know whether there are specific subgroups of patients (eg, those with moderate or severe emphysema) who derive the greatest benefit from its use. However, it is reasonable to add pneumoperitoneum in patients undergoing lower lobectomy or lower bilobectomy who are felt to be at high risk for the development of an important AL.

## POSTOPERATIVE MANAGEMENT OF ROUTINE ALs
### Chest Drain Suction Management

Despite the absence of high-level evidence to support the practice, surgeons have traditionally placed chest drains to −20 cm $H_2O$ suction following pulmonary resections, converting the tubes to waterseal only when there is no visible AL. It was suggested first in patients having

LVRS that placing patients' chest tubes to the traditional −20 cm $H_2O$ suction might prolong AALs.[56,57] Many surgeons performing LVRS now manage chest drains in these patients with waterseal alone when waterseal is tolerated. Proponents of this approach argue that its use has played a role in reducing morbidity and mortality following LVRS. This experience with LVRS stimulated surgeons to study whether various waterseal or reduced suction algorithms would reduce AL/PAL, without increasing adverse events, following other, non-LVRS pulmonary resections and in patients without severe emphysema (**Table 2**).

Cerfolio and colleagues[8] provided the first data showing that waterseal may be beneficial in allowing earlier sealing of AL even in patients without severe COPD. In this study, patients with AL present on the morning of POD2 after anatomic or lesser resections were randomized to remain on −20 suction (n = 15) or to waterseal (n = 18). In the waterseal group, 67% of the ALs sealed by POD3, whereas in the suction group only 7%

sealed ($P$ = .001). Twenty-two percent of patients placed to waterseal developed a pneumothorax and were thus placed back to −10 or −20 cm suction.

Marshall and colleagues[3] in 2002 published a study that evaluated a waterseal protocol that removes patients from suction immediately after leaving the operating room. This study, also including lobectomies and lesser resections, placed all 68 patients to −20 cm suction for the brief period between extubation and leaving the operating room, but patients were then randomized to waterseal versus continued −20 cm suction. Patients on waterseal who developed a pneumothorax greater than 25% were placed temporarily back to −10 cm suction, then back to waterseal if the space reduced. There was a significant reduction in AL duration (1.50 vs 3.27 days; $P$ = .05) in the waterseal group. Duration of chest drainage was not significantly reduced. There was no significant reduction in LOS (although it was shorter in the waterseal

**Table 2**
**Randomized prospective trials evaluating waterseal algorithms**

| Author | Algorithm Evaluated | N | Resections Included | CXRs Obtained to Rule Out PTX | Benefit to Waterseal | Significant Benefits |
|---|---|---|---|---|---|---|
| Cerfolio et al[8] | Waterseal on POD2 after −20 cm | 33 | Lobectomy and sublobar | Yes | Yes | Greater AL sealing by POD3 |
| Marshall et al[3] | Waterseal after −20 cm only while in OR | 68 | Lobectomy and sublobar | Yes | Yes | Reduced AL duration |
| Brunelli et al[7] | Waterseal on POD1 after −20 cm | 145 | Lobectomy | No | No | Do not recommend waterseal because of trend to increased complications |
| Brunelli et al[58] | Alternating −10 cm (night) and waterseal (day) on POD1 versus full-time waterseal after 10 cm of suction | 94 | Lobectomy | No | Yes (to alternating suction/waterseal) | Shorter tube duration, LOS, less PALs vs full-time waterseal |
| Alphonso et al[5] | Immediate waterseal | 239 | Lobectomy and sublobar | No | Yes | Recommend waterseal because no differences were found and waterseal promotes mobilization |

*Abbreviations:* CXRs, chest radiograms; LOS, length of stay; OR, operating room; PALs, prolonged air leaks; POD, postoperative day; PTX, pneumothorax.

group; $P = .18$). Twenty-seven percent of patients in the waterseal group developed a pneumothorax greater than 25%, but none of these caused clinical compromise. In follow-up, no patient had a clinically significant residual space or pleural effusion.

Brunelli and colleagues[7] found no benefit to waterseal, and a slightly higher complication rate in those placed to waterseal on POD1. These investigators randomized 145 patients with AL on POD1 to waterseal versus continued $-20$ cm suction. The study included only patients having lobectomy, in contrast to the previous 2 studies. There was no change in AAL duration or rate of PAL. There was a 31.9% cardiopulmonary complication rate in the waterseal group versus 17.8% in the suction group, but this did not reach statistical significance ($P = .056$).

There are a several ways to explain the differing results between the first Brunelli and colleagues[7] study and the studies by Cerfolio and colleagues[8] and Marshall and colleagues[3] that found a benefit to waterseal. First, it is possible that including lesser resections in the latter 2 studies led to their superior results with waterseal; it may be that waterseal is effective in lesser resections but not in lobectomies. Second, it is possible that the use of pleural tents by Brunelli and colleagues[7] in all upper and bilobectomies rendered unimportant a possible benefit of waterseal. A final factor that may partly account for the difference in results is that, in the study by Brunelli and colleagues,[7] chest radiograms were not obtained routinely after going to waterseal. It is therefore not clear whether some of the patients in the waterseal group may have developed an undocumented sizeable pneumothorax. Only 2.8% (n = 2) of the patients in the waterseal arm of this study were converted back to suction; in both patients this was due to the development of severe subcutaneous emphysema and desaturation. This result is in comparison with 27% in the Marshall and colleagues[3] study and 22% in the Cerfolio and colleagues[8] study being converted back to suction. It is thus possible that many patients in the Brunelli and colleagues[7] study were left with a large pneumothorax that might explain the failure of the suction arm to reduce AL duration and the slightly increased rate of cardiopulmonary complications.

Brunelli and colleagues[58] performed another randomized trial in lobectomy patients that showed a benefit to a version of part-time waterseal termed alternate suction compared with that of full-time waterseal. The investigators hypothesized that alternate suction, consisting of $-10$ cm suction during the nighttime and waterseal during the day, might combine the benefits of suction (pleural apposition) and waterseal (reducing the volume of AL; simplifying early ambulation). After maintaining $-10$ cm suction until the morning of POD1, 94 patients with AAL were randomized at that point to full-time waterseal versus alternate suction. The investigators found no difference in duration of AAL or rate of cardiopulmonary complications between the groups, but there was shorter chest tube duration ($P = .002$), shorter hospital stay ($P = .004$), and fewer PALs ($P = .02$) in the alternate suction group. In this study, chest radiograms were again not obtained routinely or after initial placement to waterseal, so there were likely some patients in the waterseal group who were left with an undiagnosed, sizeable pneumothorax. It is thus possible that the use of alternate suction by Brunelli and colleagues[58] served as the equivalent of the protocols of Cerfolio and colleagues[8] and Marshall and colleagues[3] of returning to $-10$ suction in the presence of a new or enlarging (Cerfolio) or greater than 25% (Marshall) pneumothorax.

Alphonso and colleagues[5] in 2004 performed a randomized trial that included patients having lobectomy and wedge resection (n = 239), and it differed from the other randomized studies in that patients were allocated to waterseal or suction ($-2$ kPa) immediately at the completion of surgery, such that the patients with waterseal never experienced suction. No difference was found between the 2 groups on a Kaplan-Meier analysis of AL duration ($P = .62$). None of the data on complications, LOS, or criteria for returning to suction, were provided in the study. Chest radiograms were obtained only on days 1, 3, and 7, so it is possible, as in the studies by Brunelli and colleagues,[7,58] that some unrecognized pneumothoraces were present in the patients with waterseal. It is possible that the absence of even an initial, brief period of suction to promote initial pleural apposition contributed to the lack of benefit seen in the waterseal group.

The data from these 5 randomized studies provides evidence that some version of reduced or part-time suction may reduce the duration of AL following pulmonary resection in most patients. However, the ideal waterseal or suction algorithm remains uncertain. Many potential algorithms (eg, continuous use of $-10$ cm of suction until cessation of AL) have never been studied. Available evidence suggests that alternate $-10$ cm of suction, or straight waterseal following a brief period (in the operating room only or overnight) of suction, are reasonable in patients with less than a large AAL. Provided that a sizeable pneumothorax, progressive subcutaneous emphysema, or clinical deterioration does not develop, waterseal could be maintained until chest tube removal. Optimal management with a straight suction protocol mandates a chest radiogram after being placed to waterseal. These protocols are less likely to be successful in patients with substantial restrictive lung disease, for whom complete reexpansion without suction is unlikely, and in cases with increased risk of postoperative bleeding, for which tube patency may be critical. In those situations, waterseal or reduced suction algorithms may be contraindicated.

One retrospective study addressing the use of waterseal strategies sheds further light on an important aspect of the topic. This retrospective analysis of a prospective database by Cerfolio and colleagues[21] was designed establish whether waterseal was safe and effective in patients with an AL and a pneumothorax. Of 86 such patients, 16% failed waterseal because of increasing subcutaneous emphysema or expanding, symptomatic pneumothorax. Multivariate analysis suggested that leak greater than or equal to 3 in the AL classification of Cerfolio and colleagues[8] and pneumothorax greater than 8 cm in size predicted failure of waterseal.

## POSTOPERATIVE MANAGEMENT OF PALs

It is rare that aggressive reinterventions are required to treat PALs. In several published series including more than 100 patients with PALs, the incidence of reoperation was less than 2%.[1–7] The most common treatment of PALs is watchful waiting with continued chest drainage. More than 90% of PALs stop within several weeks following operation with this form of management alone.

With continuing pressure to minimize resource use, strategies have evolved that allow treatment of PAL in the outpatient setting. These strategies involve using a one-way valve attached to the chest drain and regular outpatient visits to monitor cessation of the AAL.[9,59–62] A valved, outpatient system such as a Heimlich valve can only be considered in patients who have no more than a small, stable, asymptomatic pneumothorax on waterseal. Portable, closed one-way egress devices[63] are likely to be equally effective but have not been as well studied in this setting.

There are a combined 148 patients described within the 6 publications that report results of outpatient, one-way valves for PAL. Of these patients, all but 5 (3.4%) had their leak successfully managed in this manner. Three patients (2.0%) were readmitted with increasing pneumothorax or subcutaneous air leading to a change in therapy, and 3 patients developed infectious problems; none requiring reoperation. Only 1 of

the publications describing the use of Heimlich valves describes concurrent oral antibiotics while the tube remains in place.[9] However, the authors believe that the disadvantage of oral antibiotic coverage of skin flora while a Heimlich is in place is outweighed by its potential advantage.

It is common to have a patient with a Heimlich valve or other portable, one-way device in place who shows persistent evacuation of a few bubbles from the drain when coughing but who remains without leak on tidal breathing. Kato and colleagues[64] reported 6 patients with this sort of AL and all had at least some degree of residual postresectional pleural space. In 4 of these patients the tube thoracostomy was clamped, and 3 of the 4 had the drain successfully removed 3 to 5 days after clamping. In the remaining 2 patients, the tube was successfully removed without a trial of test clamping at 11 and 21 days after the operation. Kirschner[65] described a similar approach in an undisclosed number of patients with PAL beyond the first postoperative week. He coined the term provocative clamping. Cerfolio and colleagues[9] reported 9 patients with persistent ALs after 2 weeks of outpatient management with a Heimlich valve in whom they performed provocative clamping. All had successful tube removal without subsequent complication.

If a period of watchful waiting is unsuccessful in treating PALs, one must consider active interventions to mechanically seal the site of leak. Several methods to accomplish pleurodesis have some support in the literature. The instillation of sclerosing materials into the pleural space through the thoracostomy tube may promote symphysis of visceral and parietal pleura and leak closure. Tetracycline/doxycycline and talc are effective for pleurodesis in some cases.[66,67] The potential for microscopic contamination of the pleural space after a prolonged period with a Heimlich valve mitigates against the routine use of a foreign body such as talc. An antibiotic such as doxycycline may thus be preferable for pleurodesis in this scenario.

Autologous blood patch is another nonsurgical option to treat prolonged or persistent ALs following operation or spontaneous pneumothorax.[68–73] Blood-patch pleurodesis involves the instillation of autologous blood into the pleural space through a chest catheter. It is simple, relatively painless, and often effective, but some information suggests that blood-patch pleurodesis may also carry an increased risk of intrathoracic infection.[72,73] It may be that the infection rate will be higher if the blood patch is used after a portable, valved device has been in place for some weeks.

Invasive procedures are indicated to treat PALs if more conservative measures like watchful waiting, chemical pleurodesis, or blood-patch pleurodesis fail. Some patients may not be candidates for instillation of materials through the thoracostomy tube. Pneumoperitoneum instilled via a transabdominal catheter has been reported to be effective in some cases.[74,75] Surgical options to accomplish pleural symphysis or control the source of an AAL include video-assisted thoracoscopic surgery (VATS) with parenchymal stapling, VATS with chemical pleurodesis, VATS with pleural abrasion,[76,77] VATS with application of topical sealants,[78,79] and the less well-supported use of VATS with laser sealing of the site of leak.[80] These procedures should ideally be performed promptly after it is clear that bedside pleurodesis has failed, so that an evolving partial pleurodesis does not complicate the operation. Tissue flaps including omental or muscle flaps placed at rethoracotomy can also be used to obliterate the pleural space in patients with incomplete lung expansion and residual ALs.[81] However, most of the published experience with these flaps involves treatment of true bronchopleural fistulas and not AALs.[82–85]

Some support for recently introduced bronchoscopic techniques also exists in the literature, but with limited levels of evidence. Ferguson and colleagues,[86] for example, suggest that an endobronchial artificial valve may limit PALs after lung volume reduction procedures.

Other rarely used interventions have been reported to successfully treat PAL in special circumstances. For example, patients with PALs from incompletely resected pulmonary malignancy may benefit from radiation therapy to treat the malignancy and limit the AL.[87] For patients who are intubated and whose PAL causes significant inspiratory volume loss, a double-lumen endotracheal tube with single-lung ventilation may help to seal the leak and allow adequate ventilation.[88] Another technique described for PAL is the use of tissue expanders to create an artificial symphysis between the tissue expander and the visceral pleura.[89]

In summary, prolonged alveolar AALs will usually stop with conservative therapy alone that most appropriately consists of outpatient management with a Heimlich valve. Gradual escalation of therapy is indicated after a period of a few weeks, and there is a spectrum of choices for therapy that includes sclerosing agents instilled via tube thoracostomy, recently propose bronchoscopic interventions, VATS or thoracotomy for direct repair of the leak site or pleurodesis, or tissue flap transposition. Of the more aggressive interventions described for treatment of PALs, one technique cannot be recommended in preference to another based on the available evidence. Clinical judgment, taking into consideration individual patient factors and knowledge of all available options, offers the best solution to complex PAL management.

## ACKNOWLEDGMENTS

The authors would like to acknowledge Donna Minagawa for technical help with the manuscript.

## REFERENCES

1. Antanavicius G, Lamb J, Papasavas P, et al. Initial chest tube management after pulmonary resection. Am Surg 2005;71:416–9.
2. Okamoto J, Okamoto T, Fukuyama Y, et al. The use of a water seal to manage air leaks after a pulmonary lobectomy: a retrospective study. Ann Thorac Cardiovasc Surg 2006;12:242–4.
3. Marshall MB, Deeb ME, Bleier JI, et al. Suction vs water seal after pulmonary resection: a randomized prospective study. Chest 2002;121:831–5.
4. Okereke I, Murthy SC, Alster JM, et al. Characterization and importance of air leak after lobectomy. Ann Thorac Surg 2005;79:1167–73.
5. Alphonso N, Tan C, Utley M, et al. A prospective randomized controlled trial of suction versus nonsuction to the under-water seal drains following lung resection. Eur J Cardiothorac Surg 2005;27:391–4.
6. Cerfolio RJ, Tummala RP, Holman WL, et al. A prospective algorithm for the management of air leaks after pulmonary resection. Ann Thorac Surg 1998;66:1726–31.
7. Brunelli A, Monteverde M, Borri A, et al. Comparison of water seal and suction after pulmonary lobectomy: a prospective, randomized trial. Ann Thorac Surg 2004;77:1932–7 [discussion: 1937].
8. Cerfolio RJ, Bass C, Katholi CR. Prospective randomized trial compares suction versus water seal for air leaks. Ann Thorac Surg 2001;71:1613–7.
9. Cerfolio RJ, Bass CS, Pask AH, et al. Predictors and treatment of persistent air leaks. Ann Thorac Surg 2002;73:1727–30 [discussion: 1730–1].
10. DeCamp MM, Blackstone EH, Naunheim KS, et al. Patient and surgical factors influencing air leak after lung volume reduction surgery: lessons learned from the National Emphysema Treatment Trial. Ann Thorac Surg 2006;82:197–206 [discussion: 206–7].
11. Varela G, Jimenez MF, Novoa N, et al. Estimating hospital costs attributable to prolonged air leak in pulmonary lobectomy. Eur J Cardiothorac Surg 2005;27:329–33.
12. Bardell T, Petsikas D. What keeps postpulmonary resection patients in hospital? Can Respir J 2003; 10:86–9.

13. Linden PA, Bueno R, Colson YL, et al. Lung resection in patients with preoperative FEV$_1$ < 35% predicted. Chest 2005;127:1984–90.

14. Zegdi R, Azorin J, Tremblay B, et al. Videothoracoscopic lung biopsy in diffuse infiltrative lung diseases: a 5-year surgical experience. Ann Thorac Surg 1998;66:1170–3.

15. Kreider ME, Hansen-Flaschen J, Ahmad NN, et al. Complications of video-assisted thoracoscopic lung biopsy in patients with interstitial lung disease. Ann Thorac Surg 2007;83:1140–4.

16. Cho MH, Malhotra A, Donahue DM, et al. Mechanical ventilation and air leaks after lung biopsy for acute respiratory distress syndrome. Ann Thorac Surg 2006;82:261–6.

17. Brunelli A, Xiume F, Al Refai M, et al. Air leaks after lobectomy increase the risk of empyema but not of cardiopulmonary complications: a case-matched analysis. Chest 2006;130:1150–6.

18. Irshad K, Feldman LS, Chu VF, et al. Causes of increased length of hospitalization on a general thoracic surgery service: a prospective observational study. Can J Surg 2002;45:264–8.

19. Brunelli A, Moteverde M, Borri A, et al. Predictors of prolonged air leak after pulmonary lobectomy. Ann Thorac Surg 2004;77:1205–10.

20. Stolz AJ, Schutzner J, Lischke R, et al. Predictors of prolonged air leak following pulmonary lobectomy. Eur J Cardiothorac Surg 2005;27:334–6.

21. Cerfolio RJ, Bryant AS, Singh S, et al. The management of chest tubes in patients with a pneumothorax and an air leak after pulmonary resection. Chest 2005;128:816–20.

22. Cerfolio RJ, Bryant AS. The benefits of continuous and digital air leak assessment after elective pulmonary resection: a prospective study. Ann Thorac Surg 2008;86:396–401.

23. Varela G, Jimemnez MF, Novoa NM, et al. Postoperative chest tube management: measuring leaks using an electronic device decreases variability in clinical practice. Eur J Cardiothorac Surg 2006;35:28–31.

24. Brunelli A, Salati M, Refai M, et al. Evaluation of a new chest tube removal protocol using direct air leak monitoring after lobectomy: a prospective randomized trial. Eur J Cardiothorac Surg 2010;37(1):56–60.

25. Cooper JD. Technique to reduce air leaks after resection of emphysematous lung. Ann Thorac Surg 1994;57:1038–9.

26. Vaughn CC, Wolner E, Dahan M, et al. Prevention of air leaks after pulmonary wedge resection. Ann Thorac Surg 1997;63:864–6.

27. Thomas P, Massard G, Porte H, et al. A new bioabsorbable sleeve for lung staple-line reinforcement (FOREseal): report of a three-center phase II clinical trial. Eur J Cardiothorac Surg 2006;29:880–5.

28. Hazelrigg SR, Boley TM, Naunheim KS, et al. Effect of bovine pericardial strips on air leak after stapled pulmonary resection. Ann Thorac Surg 1997;63:1573–5.

29. Stammberger U, Klopotko W, Stamatis G, et al. Buttressing the staple line in lung volume reduction surgery: a randomized three-center study. Ann Thorac Surg 2000;70:1820–5.

30. Miller JI Jr, Landreneau RJ, Wright CE, et al. A comparative study of buttressed versus nonbuttressed staple line in pulmonary resections. Ann Thorac Surg 2001;71:319–22 [discussion: 323].

31. Venuta F, Rendina EA, De Giacomo T, et al. Technique to reduce air leaks after pulmonary lobectomy. Eur J Cardiothorac Surg 1998;13:361–4.

32. Serra-Mitjans M, Belda-Sanchis J, Rami-Porta R. Surgical sealant for preventing air leaks after pulmonary resections in patients with lung cancer. Cochrane Database Syst Rev 2005;3:CD003051.

33. Tambiah J, Rawlins R, Robb D, et al. Can tissue adhesives and glues significantly reduce the incidence and length of postoperative air leaks in patients having lung resections? Interact Cardiovasc Thorac Surg 2007;6:529–33.

34. Fabian T, Federico JA, Ponn RB. Fibrin glue in pulmonary resection: a prospective, randomized, blinded study. Ann Thorac Surg 2003;75:1587–92.

35. Fleisher AG, Evans KG, Nelems B, et al. Effect of routine fibrin glue use on the duration of air leaks after lobectomy. Ann Thorac Surg 1990;49:133–4.

36. Wong K, Goldstraw P. Effect of fibrin glue in the reduction of postthoracotomy alveolar air leak. Ann Thorac Surg 1997;64:979–81.

37. Mouritzen C, Dromer M, Keinecke HO. The effect of fibrin glueing to seal bronchial and alveolar leakages after pulmonary resections and decortications. Eur J Cardiothorac Surg 1993;7:75–80.

38. Wurtz A, Chambon JP, Sobecki L, et al. [Use of a biological glue in partial pulmonary excision surgery. Results of a controlled trial in 50 patients]. Ann Chir 1991;45:719–23 [in French].

39. Porte HL, Jany T, Akkad R, et al. Randomized controlled trial of a synthetic sealant for preventing alveolar air leaks after lobectomy. Ann Thorac Surg 2001;71:1618–22.

40. Macchiarini P, Wain J, Almy S, et al. Experimental and clinical evaluation of a new synthetic, absorbable sealant to reduce air leaks in thoracic operations. J Thorac Cardiovasc Surg 1999;117:751–8.

41. Wain JC, Kaiser LR, Johnstone DW, et al. Trial of a novel synthetic sealant in preventing air leaks after lung resection. Ann Thorac Surg 2001;71:1623–8 [discussion: 1628–9].

42. Allen MS, Wood DE, Hawkinson RW, et al. Prospective randomized study evaluating a biodegradable polymeric sealant for sealing intraoperative air leaks that occur during pulmonary resection. Ann Thorac Surg 2004;77:1792–801.

43. Wurtz A, Gambiez L, Chambon J, et al. Evaluation de l'efficacité d'une colle de fibrine en chirurgie d'exérèse pulmonaire partielle. Résultats d'un nouvel essai contrôlé chez 50 malades. Lyon Chir 1992;88:368–71 [in French].

44. Lang G, Csekeo A, Stamatis G, et al. Efficacy and safety of topical application of human fibrinogen/thrombin-coated collagen patch (TachoComb) for treatment of air leakage after standard lobectomy. Eur J Cardiothorac Surg 2004;25:160–6.

45. D'Andrilli A, Andreetti C, Ibrahim M, et al. A prospective randomized study to assess the efficacy of a surgical sealant to treat air leaks in lung surgery. Eur J Cardiothorac Surg 2009;35(5):817–20 [discussion: 820–1].

46. Rena O, Papalia E, Mineo TC, et al. Air-leak management after upper lobectomy in patients with fused fissure and chronic obstructive pulmonary disease: a pilot trial comparing sealant and standard treatment. Interact Cardiovasc Thorac Surg 2009;9(6):973–7.

47. Anegg U, Lindenmann J, Matzi V, et al. Efficiency of fleece-bound sealing (TachoSil) of air leaks in lung surgery: a prospective randomised trial. Eur J Cardiothorac Surg 2007;31(2):198–202.

48. Belboul A, Dernevik L, Aljassim O, et al. The effect of autologous fibrin sealant (Vivostat) on morbidity after pulmonary lobectomy: a prospective randomised, blinded study. Eur J Cardiothorac Surg 2004;26:1187–91.

49. Moser C, Opitz I, Zhai W, et al. Autologous fibrin sealant reduces the incidence of prolonged air leak and duration of chest tube drainage after lung volume reduction surgery: a prospective randomized blinded study. J Thorac Cardiovasc Surg 2008;136(4):843–9.

50. Tansley P, Al-Mulhim F, Lim E, et al. A prospective, randomized, controlled trial of the effectiveness of BioGlue in treating alveolar air leaks. J Thorac Cardiovasc Surg 2006;132:105–12.

51. Brunelli A, Al Refai M, Monteverde M, et al. Pleural tent after upper lobectomy: a randomized study of efficacy and duration of effect. Ann Thorac Surg 2002;74:1958–62.

52. Okur E, Kir A, Halezeroglu S, et al. Pleural tenting following upper lobectomies or bilobectomies of the lung to prevent residual air space and prolonged air leak. Eur J Cardiothorac Surg 2001;20:1012–5.

53. Robinson LA, Preksto D. Pleural tenting during upper lobectomy decreases chest tube time and total hospitalization days. J Thorac Cardiovasc Surg 1998;115:319–26 [discussion: 326–7].

54. Toker A, Dilege S, Tanju S, et al. Perioperative pneumoperitoneum after lobectomy – bilobectomy operations for lung cancer: a prospective study. Thorac Cardiovasc Surg 2003;51:93–6.

55. Cerfolio RJ, Holman WL, Katholi CR. Pneumoperitoneum after concomitant resection of the right middle and lower lobes (bilobectomy). Ann Thorac Surg 2000;70:942–6 [discussion: 946–7].

56. Cooper JD, Patterson GA, Sundaresan RS, et al. Results of 150 consecutive bilateral lung volume reduction procedures in patients with severe emphysema. J Thorac Cardiovasc Surg 1996;112:1319–29 [discussion: 1329–30].

57. Cooper JD, Patterson GA. Lung-volume reduction surgery for severe emphysema. Chest Surg Clin N Am 1995;5:815–31.

58. Brunelli A, Sabbatini A, Xiume F, et al. Alternate suction reduces prolonged air leak after pulmonary lobectomy: a randomized comparison versus water seal. Ann Thorac Surg 2005;80:1052–5.

59. McKenna RJ Jr, Fischel RJ, Brenner M, et al. Use of the Heimlich valve to shorten hospital stay after lung reduction surgery for emphysema. Ann Thorac Surg 1996;61:1115–7.

60. Ponn RB, Silverman HJ, Federico JA. Outpatient chest tube management. Ann Thorac Surg 1997;64:1437–40.

61. McKenna RJ, Mahtabifard A, Pickens A, et al. Fast-tracking after video-assisted thoracoscopic surgery lobectomy, segmentectomy, and pneumonectomy. Ann Thorac Surg 2007;84:1663–7.

62. McManus KG, Spence GM, McGuigan JA. Outpatient chest tubes. Ann Thorac Surg 1998;66:299–300.

63. Rieger KM, Wroblewski HA, Brooks JA, et al. Postoperative outpatient chest tube management: initial experience with a new portable system. Ann Thorac Surg 2007;84:630–2.

64. Kato R, Kobayashi T, Watanabe M, et al. Can the chest tube draining the pleural cavity with persistent air leakage be removed? Thorac Cardiovasc Surg 1992;40:292–6.

65. Kirschner PA. "Provocative clamping" and removal of chest tubes despite persistent air leak. Ann Thorac Surg 1992;53:740–1.

66. Read CA, Reddy VD, O'Mara TE, et al. Doxycycline pleurodesis for pneumothorax in patients with AIDS. Chest 1994;105:823–5.

67. Kilic D, Findikcioglu A, Hatipoglu A. A different application method of talc pleurodesis for the treatment of persistent air leak. ANZ J Surg 2006;76:754–6.

68. Droghetti A, Schiavini A, Muriana P, et al. Autologous blood patch in persistent air leaks after pulmonary resection. J Thorac Cardiovasc Surg 2006;132:556–9.

69. Shackcloth MJ, Poullis M, Jackson M, et al. Intrapleural instillation of autologous blood in the treatment of prolonged air leak after lobectomy: a prospective randomized controlled trial. Ann Thorac Surg 2006;82:1052–6.

70. Yokomise H, Satoh K, Ohno N, et al. Autoblood plus OK432 pleurodesis with open drainage for persistent air leak after lobectomy. Ann Thorac Surg 1998;65:563–5.

71. Dumire R, Crabbe MM, Mappin FG, et al. Autologous "blood patch" pleurodesis for persistent pulmonary air leak. Chest 1992;101:64–6.

72. Cagirici U, Sahin B, Cakan A, et al. Autologous blood patch pleurodesis in spontaneous pneumothorax with persistent air leak. Scand Cardiovasc J 1998;32:75–8.

73. Lang-Lazdunski L, Coonar AS. A prospective study of autologous 'blood patch' pleurodesis for persistent air leak after pulmonary resection. Eur J Cardiothorac Surg 2004;26:897–900.

74. De Giacomo T, Rendina EA, Venuta F, et al. Pneumoperitoneum for the management of pleural air space problems associated with major pulmonary resections. Ann Thorac Surg 2001;72:1716–9.

75. Handy JR Jr, Judson MA, Zellner JL. Pneumoperitoneum to treat air leaks and spaces after a lung volume reduction operation. Ann Thorac Surg 1997;64:1803–5.

76. Suter M, Bettschart V, Vandoni RE, et al. Thoracoscopic pleurodesis for prolonged (or intractable) air leak after lung resection. Eur J Cardiothorac Surg 1997;12:160–1.

77. Torre M, Grassi M, Nerli FP, et al. Nd-YAG laser pleurodesis via thoracoscopy. Endoscopic therapy in spontaneous pneumothorax Nd-YAG laser pleurodesis. Chest 1994;106:338–41.

78. Carrillo EH, Kozloff M, Saridakis A, et al. Thoracoscopic application of a topical sealant for the management of persistent posttraumatic pneumothorax. J Trauma 2006;60:111–4.

79. Thistlethwaite PA, Luketich JD, Ferson PF, et al. Ablation of persistent air leaks after thoracic procedures with fibrin sealant. Ann Thorac Surg 1999;67:575–7.

80. Sharpe DA, Dixon C, Moghissi K. Thoracoscopic use of laser in intractable pneumothorax. Eur J Cardiothorac Surg 1994;8:34–6.

81. Nonami Y, Ogoshi S. Omentopexy for empyema due to lung fistula following lobectomy. A case report. J Cardiovasc Surg (Torino) 1998;39:695–6.

82. Backhus LM, Sievers EM, Schenkel FA, et al. Pleural space problems after living lobar transplantation. J Heart Lung Transplant 2005;24:2086–90.

83. Colwell AS, Mentzer SJ, Vargas SO, et al. The role of muscle flaps in pulmonary aspergillosis. Plast Reconstr Surg 2003;111:1147–50.

84. Francel TJ, Lee GW, Mackinnon SE, et al. Treatment of long-standing thoracostoma and bronchopleural fistula without pulmonary resection in high risk patients. Plast Reconstr Surg 1997;99:1046–53.

85. Hammond DC, Fisher J, Meland NB. Intrathoracic free flaps. Plast Reconstr Surg 1993;91:1259–64.

86. Ferguson JS, Sprenger K, Van Natta T. Closure of a bronchopleural fistula using bronchoscopic placement of an endobronchial valve designed for the treatment of emphysema. Chest 2006;129:479–81.

87. Ong YE, Sheth A, Simmonds NJ, et al. Radiotherapy: a novel treatment for pneumothorax. Eur Respir J 2006;27:427–9.

88. Rankin N, Day AC, Crone PD. Traumatic massive air leak treated with prolonged double lumen intubation and high frequency ventilation: case report. J Trauma 1994;36:428–9.

89. Sakamaki Y, Kido T, Fujiwara T, et al. A novel procedure using a tissue expander for management of persistent alveolar fistula after lobectomy. Ann Thorac Surg 2005;79:2130–2.

# Index

*Note:* Page numbers of article titles are in **boldface** type.

## A

AAL. See *Alveolar air leaks.*
Air leaks
    chest drain suction management of, 441–444
    chest drainage systems for monitoring of,
       413–419
    and chest tube management, 353
    and chronic obstructive pulmonary disease, 391
    and emphysema, 391, 393–394
    and endobronchial one-way valves, 394
    evidence-based suggestions for management of,
       435–445
    grading system for, 436–437
    incidence of, 436
    intraoperative management of, 437–441
    and lobectomy, 435–438, 441–443
    and lung volume reduction surgery, 391, 394
    management of, 401–403
    permanent, 391–394
    persistent, 403
    and pleural drain management, 391–392
    and pleural tent, 440–441
    and pleurodesis, 393
    and pneumoperitoneum, 393–394
    postoperative management of, 441
    and prevention of residual air spaces,
       371–374
    and reoperation, 394
    risk factors after lung resection, 359–363
    risk factors for, 436
    significance of, 436
    and thoracostomy tube, 444–445
    and use of sealants and buttressing material,
       377–387
Air spaces
    intraoperative options for management of, 372
    intraoperative prevention of, 371–374
Alveolar air leaks, 435–445
    and bronchopleural fistula, 435, 445
    and pneumoperitoneum, 441
    and pneumothorax, 436–437, 442–444
    and sealants, 438–440
Ambulatory pleural drainage, 421–425
    devices available for, 424
    and Heimlich valves, 422, 424–425
    reported experiences of, 422

## B

Barotrauma. See *Air leaks.*
Biologic sealants, 377–381
BPF. See *Bronchopleural fistula.*
Bronchopleural fistula
    and alveolar air leaks, 435, 445
Buttressing material
    staple-line, 385–387

## C

Chest drainage systems
    digital pleural, 413–417
    for monitoring air leaks, 413–419
    portable, 414, 421–425
Chest tubes
    active suction compared with passive suction,
       400–401
    and air leak evaluation, 401
    and air leaks, 353, 360–362
    and chest x-rays, 404
    and evidence-based medicine, 401
    and high-volume drainage, 404
    history of, 399
    and hydrothorax, 353–354
    management after pulmonary resection, 399–404
    outpatient management of, 403–404, 423
    portable chest drainage systems for outpatient
       management of, 421–425
    and water seal suction, 399–404
Chest wall
    muscles, 373
    osteotendinous, 374
Chest wall muscles
    and prevention of residual air spaces, 373
Chest x-rays
    and chest tubes, 404
Chronic obstructive pulmonary disease
    and permanent air leaks, 391
    and prolonged air leaks, 436
Collagen fleece-bound fibrin sealants, 383–385
    clinical evidence regarding, 383–385
    complications of, 385
    experimental evidence regarding, 383
    and findings in randomized clinical trials, 384
    and pulmonary resection, 383–385

Thorac Surg Clin 20 (2010) 449–452
doi:10.1016/S1547-4127(10)00101-5
1547-4127/10/$ – see front matter © 2010 Elsevier Inc. All rights reserved.

thoracic.theclinics.com

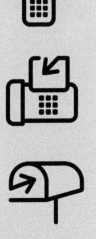